INSOURCED

Dr. Kate Tulenko

INSOURCED

How Importing Jobs Impacts the Healthcare Crisis Here and Abroad

Dartmouth College Press
Hanover, New Hampshire

DARTMOUTH COLLEGE PRESS
An imprint of University Press of New England
www.upne.com

Manufactured in the United States of America
Designed by Eric M. Brooks
Typeset in Fresco Plus Pro and Officina Sans
by Passumpsic Publishing

University Press of New England is a member of the Green Press Initiative. The paper used in this book meets their minimum requirement for recycled paper.

Library of Congress Cataloging-in-Publication Data
Tulenko, Kate.
Insourced: how importing jobs impacts the healthcare crisis here and abroad / Kate Tulenko.
p.; cm.
Includes bibliographical references.
ISBN 978-1-61168-227-4 (cloth: alk. paper)—
ISBN 978-1-61168-268-7 (ebook)
I. Title. [DNLM: 1. Foreign Professional Personnel—supply & distribution—United States.
2. Developing Countries—United States.
3. Health Manpower—trends—United States.
4. Health Personnel—education—United States.
5. Medically Underserved Area—United States. W 76]
610.73'7069091724—dc23 2011047068

5 4 3 2 1

To my husband, Ken Heyman,

and my daughters, Helena and Freya,

for all their love, support, and lonely Saturdays,

which made this book possible.

Contents

Foreword *by Laurie Garrett* / ix

Preface / xiii

Acknowledgments / xxv

Introduction / 1

1 Shortage in the Land of Abundance / 10

2 How the United States Created Its Healthcare-Workforce Problem / 40

3 The Path to America / 66

4 The Damage Done / 91

5 The Fox and the Hydra
Failed Attempts to Address Insourcing / 116

6 Successful Efforts to Curb Insourcing / 138

7 The Way Forward / 150

Notes / 181

Index / 197

Foreword

It's hard to imagine any realistic conversation about global health that doesn't begin with the question: "Where are the health-care workers?" In 2004 Lincoln Chen and Tim Evans told us[1] that the world was facing a profound deficit of some 4.3 million health professionals; for sub-Saharan Africa alone, the deficit was 1 million.

Since then the pressures on the global health labor force have only increased, and training of doctors, nurses, dentists, pharmacists, lab technicians, midwives, medical supplies experts, hospital administrators, optometrists, and every other type of health professional remains woefully inadequate.

The most acute shortages of skilled health personnel are in countries facing the gravest public health challenges. For example, in rural Mozambique, where HIV rates exceed 10% of the adult population and famine shadows the people with shocking regularity, the few physicians available have a patient load of 6,496 patients per MD, about twenty times the burden doctors face in the capital city of Maputo.[2] Any initiative to improve the well-being of Mozambique's largely rural population must begin by asking who will actually implement programs of mass immunization, HIV testing, prenatal care, safe drinking water, or malaria prevention.

The spectacular boom in global health financing between 2002 and 2009, jumping from roughly $5.6 billion to more than $20 billion, allowed the world to dream *big*: Eradicate malaria, provide universal access to HIV treatment, stop the spread of drug-resistant tuberculosis, and bring maternal mortality rates in poor countries down to the levels found in North America. But as ambitious programs were rolled out, often in great haste, implementers realized the scale of the healthcare worker crisis. A mad scramble ensued, as skilled professionals were wooed away from their often dismal government jobs to work on externally supported health initiatives.

The brain drain from one sector to another within countries might have been tolerable if it had not occurred amid two larger global forces: gross underpayment of public sector health workers, and pull from wealthy countries.

A sad truism is that highly skilled physicians and nurses in most countries of the developing world and even emerging market nations can earn more money driving taxis or selling cars than they can by performing trauma surgery or treating malarial encephalitis. In Dr. Kate Tulenko's book you will read the numbers—a state of affairs increasingly seen in rich countries, as well. A newly minted American physician now often faces decades of student loan payments, the interest and duration of which cannot be shortened by accepting a position in a rural county hospital or inner city clinic. All over the world the basic economics of salaries and cost of living drive skilled professionals either out of the health field entirely or else toward practices in populations that are already relatively well served. To put it crassly, the economic model favors Beverly Hills plastic surgeons over primary care physicians in rural Iowa.

A former U.S. presidential candidate named Ross Perot famously referred to "that giant sucking sound" of American jobs allegedly sucked away to Mexico. In truth the massive "sucking sound" is that of health professionals enticed to abandon their home countries for higher paying positions in wealthier nations. As Tulenko details in this book, the lure often proves less glamorous or rewarding than immigrating healthcare workers expect. But the numbers of those sucked away from their home countries to fill the ranks of healthcare workers elsewhere are enormous. In Lesotho doctors told me of losing nurses to Botswana; the Botswana losses are to South Africa. Walk the halls of England's National Health Service and hear nurses speaking Zulu and Xhosa—evidence that South Africa is losing personnel to wealthier Commonwealth countries.

Years ago I was asked to testify on the healthcare worker crisis before the Senate Foreign Relations Committee. I told the committee members that it was unconscionable that the United States was actively recruiting healthcare workers from the Caribbean, Mexico, the Philippines, India, and other poorer countries, while also refusing to provide serious funds to support domestic schools of nursing, dentistry, and medicine. As unemployment rose inside the United States, many laid-off workers were encouraged to go back to school to obtain health sector training. Yet an array of factors conspired against any hope that these jobless workers could fill America's yawning gap in health professionals. As detailed in this book, one such factor is inadequate funding for professors, resulting in students' inability to obtain sufficient training to pass licensing examinations. Another concerns compensation: many hospitals and insurance schemes reimburse physicians and other health professionals so poorly that newly minted workers swiftly discern that their lifestyles will be well below expectations, especially during the years of labor required to pay off student loans.

The worldwide demographic shift toward older populations signifies still harsher pressures on healthcare systems, especially for labor-intensive chronic and geriatric care. This shift is felt powerfully in Europe, Japan, China, North America, and pockets of populations all over the world. So the enormous unfilled current demand for skilled healthcare workers will only worsen with time, and with population aging.

Many solutions suggest themselves. Some possibilities are detailed by Dr. Tulenko in this book. No nation or population is without need for health talent; therefore, no country can be spared the pressure to find answers, innovate, and ultimately rethink the structure and personnel allotment of its health system.

Laurie Garrett
Senior Fellow for Global Health,
Council on Foreign Relations
Author of Betrayal of Trust: The Collapse of Global Public Health

Notes

1 http://www.who.int/hrh/documents/JLi_hrh_report.pdf; Lincoln C. Chen, Tim Evans, and Jacob Silberberg, *Human Resources for Health: Overcoming the Crisis* (Cambridge, Mass.: Global Equity Initiative, 2004).

2 William McGreevey, Carlos Avila, and Maria Punchak, *Assessment Paper: Strengthening Health Systems* (ReThink HIV, Copenhagen Consensus Center, 2011).

Preface

In developing countries, a child dies every four seconds. A major reason for such needless death is the lack of enough doctors, nurses, and other healthcare providers to prevent and treat illness. The global healthcare-worker shortage has been called the greatest humanitarian crisis of our time because it cuts across every crisis, from disease outbreaks to national disasters to wars, and hamstrings our ability to respond. As a mother, a pediatrician, and a health-policy expert, I feel deeply the urgent need to address this issue.

During my time at the World Bank, I saw people out of work in the US while good jobs sat empty in their communities. I saw health workers being imported from countries that could ill afford to lose them. But no one seemed to be making the connection between the two problems and offering solutions. Many wealthy countries have their own shortage of healthcare workers, and rather than paying to train their own young people to work in these fields, these countries, led by the United States, are importing healthcare workers from poor countries. This practice has severely distorted and damaged the healthcare systems in those countries and has created perverse incentives to produce healthcare workers for export rather than to meet the needs of their own people.

Concentrating on a short-term solution, the United States and other wealthy countries are failing to address the reasons they do not have enough healthcare workers and ignoring the damage they are doing both at home and abroad. So I have pursued the topic by researching and writing this book during vacation time, early-morning writing sessions, caffeinated evenings, and an extended maternity leave.

My first exposure to health-workforce issues came as a student at the Johns Hopkins School of Public Health. My two advisers were Dr. Tim Baker, one of the giants of health-workforce planning, and Dr. Richard Morrow, a leader in introducing quality-assurance management and team efficiency into the field of public health. Both of them taught me that beyond and often more important than the science of medicine was the healthcare team: the actual people and personalities who delivered healthcare.

My first opportunity to work formally on health-workforce issues came right after I graduated from Johns Hopkins University School of Medicine, in Baltimore, in 1999. I was doing my residency at Children's National Medical Center, a top-ranked pediatric hospital in Washington, DC. To improve the quality and cost-effectiveness of its care, the hospital had recently added several types of healthcare workers to its staff teams. For example, phlebotomists, who are technicians specialized in drawing blood, now drew most of the blood samples for lab tests, which saved the pediatric residents hours of time they could spend treating patients. Phlebotomists have been shown to be at least as effective in drawing blood as physicians, and their wages are less than residents' wages, so there were cost savings, too.

At the hospital, X-ray and lab technicians had taken on very important tasks that freed up the more expensive time of the radiologists and pathologists. Physician assistants and nurse practitioners provided high-quality care that allowed the physicians to focus on more complicated aspects of diagnosis and treatment. Advanced-practice nurses, with several years of additional training in a subspecialty, such as pediatric cardiology, enabled the pediatric cardiologists to care more effectively for more patients. Because advanced-practice nurses specialize, they have more in-depth knowledge in their specialty area than the general pediatric residents, who practice just a few months of pediatric cardiology each year.

I had noticed the impressive ways in which the new healthcare workers had increased productivity at the hospital. So naturally, when a seat for a resident opened on the Expanded-Roles Committee (which advised on how nonphysician healthcare workers could be used to provide higher-quality, more cost-effective care), I jumped at the chance.

While I was completing my clinical training, I was also pursuing my other passion: global health. Foreign cultures have been a particular interest of mine ever since I was a child and found a book on Mayan culture in my parents' library. The notion of a people who had mapped the skies centuries before anyone in a Western culture, yet whose written language consisted of pictures rather than letters, fascinated me. Specializing in the field of global health—which seeks to improve the health of people all over the world, in different types of cultures, especially those in developing countries—gave me a way to combine my love of anthropology and my love of medicine.

As a resident, I served on the American Academy of Pediatrics' Section on International Child Health, which works to improve the health of children in developing countries. The vast majority of child deaths are in developing countries, and about half of those deaths occur in Africa. In many African countries, one out of four children dies before his or her fifth birthday. That is 25 percent of all the children born in those countries! In the United States, only one in 1,600 children dies before his or her fifth birthday, and most of these deaths are due to accidents. Most newborn deaths in the United States are due to unpreventable birth defects or severe prematurity, for which even the most advanced medicine can offer little help. In my entire US pediatric career, I have had just four patients die: a teenager with an inherited disease of the heart muscle, a teen with chronic bowel disease, a teenage member of a Middle Eastern royal family who had advanced lymphoma, and a micro-preemie with multiple birth defects.

In developing countries, the most common causes of child death include birth injuries, diarrhea, pneumonia, malaria, and vaccine-preventable diseases. In countries such as India, Ethiopia, and Nigeria, many infants die shortly after they are born, simply because there are too few physicians and midwives to attend all the deliveries and address common newborn complications. As a result, the main global project of the American Academy of Pediatrics is Helping Babies Breathe, a program through which community-based healthcare workers are trained in basic newborn-resuscitation techniques.

It took a while to dawn on me that in both streams of my career, I was working on the same issue: the shortage of healthcare workers in developing countries *and* in the United States.

In 2002, after completing my pediatrics residency, I had an opportunity to join the World Bank. This is the United Nations agency that provides developing countries with financing and expert advice in every economic sector, from agriculture to education to transport. The World Bank is one of the largest non-government funders of healthcare programs in these countries, and joining its health team was an incredible chance to make a difference. An added benefit was that I could keep up my clinical work through weekend shifts in the Children's National Medical Center emergency room.

I entered through the World Bank's Young Professionals (YP) program. Every year, about 13,000 people apply for the 35 slots in this management-training program; it's an offer you cannot refuse. As a YP, I had the opportunity to work in several different regional healthcare units before settling down to work in the Africa health unit.

Once I started traveling frequently for the World Bank, it became difficult to schedule my shifts in the emergency room, so I started working with hospitals and clinics in underserved communities in the Washington, DC, area. These facilities often had trouble filling their permanent positions, so they were happy to have me come in on short notice on a weekend here and there. I worked much of my time at Mary's Center for Maternal and Child Health, also in Washington, DC.

Mary's Center has an interesting history. In the 1980s, as thousands of war refugees from Guatemala, El Salvador, and Nicaragua came into the United States, many joined the growing Central American communities in Washington, DC. Undocumented and without health insurance, many of the women gave birth at home, without any medical care for themselves or their babies. So many women with severe labor complications and sick children began showing up at the hospitals and clinics that the local government assisted in founding a new clinic to provide care to Spanish-speaking women and their children.

The founders knew the clinic could save money in the long term by preventing costly birth and health complications. Mary's Center is a federally qualified health center, a designation that allows it to receive special federal funds to provide care to medically underserved populations: recent immigrants, the homeless, public-housing residents, and the uninsured. But the requirement that all staff members speak Spanish and the fact that it paid less than half the going rate for physicians in the DC area meant that it was chronically short staffed. I filled in as needed, mainly on weekends and when full-time staff members weren't available.

I supplemented this with on-call work at a variety of clinics and hospitals in medically underserved communities in rural Maryland and Virginia. If you drive an hour and a half in almost any direction from Washington, DC, you find yourself in a rural community with a healthcare-worker shortage. Often, the community has just one or two pediatricians. I was delighted to work in Queen Anne's County, Maryland, in a clinic near the tiny town of Rock Hall (population 1,396), where I spent most of my childhood summers on my uncle's farm and where my cousin is the fund-raiser at the local hospital.

I also worked in Carroll Hospital Center, in Carroll County, Maryland, attending high-risk deliveries and caring for the children in the pediatrics ward. The hospital was short three pediatricians, and the lone staff pediatrician was alternating night shifts with local clinic-based pediatricians, many of whom had little experience with critically ill children. It turns out this type of substitute work is a $2 billion-a-year Band-Aid solution to the severe shortage and maldistribution of healthcare workers in the United States.[1] The other Band-Aid solution is importing tens of thousands of foreign-trained healthcare workers each year.

It's not just ultra-poor or "basket case" countries that are affected by our demand for their healthcare providers. From 2006 to 2008, during my time at the World Bank, I had the rare privilege of working in Barbados. I had to suffer through a lot of jokes and comments from my colleagues about "hardship travel" and writing reports on the beach. But it was deeply serious business. The Caribbean has the highest rates of HIV/AIDS outside Africa—Haiti, Jamaica, and the Bahamas all have HIV rates near or above 2 percent.[2]

The HIV/AIDS epidemic did more than threaten the lives of the Caribbean people; it threatened their livelihoods. Tourism is a crucial source of income for most Caribbean countries, and during the first wave of news regarding the high HIV rates in the Caribbean, some countries saw significant drops in tourist visits. That caused many officials to purposely deny or underplay the situation rather than planning an adequate response to the crisis.[3]

Barbados, however, has shown incredible leadership in openly addressing its HIV/AIDS crisis, creating special programs to prevent the spread of the disease as well as to diagnose and treat anyone on the island with HIV. Even so, the response of Barbados and the other Caribbean countries has been hindered by their healthcare-workforce shortage. We might think of the Caribbean as a sunny vacationland, but there is great poverty there; the per capita gross domestic product in Barbados and many other Caribbean nations is less than half that in the United States. Unable to pay their healthcare workers anywhere near as much as they can earn in the United States, and unable to afford the technology that makes medical practice more rewarding and intellectually stimulating, the Caribbean has seen large numbers of its doctors and nurses emigrate. One estimate is that three times as many Caribbean-educated nurses are working outside the Caribbean as in their home countries.[4]

The shortage of healthcare workers in the Caribbean is actually thought to impede the economic development of the region. The poor health of its citizens causes lost productivity and extra medical costs. Beyond that, the lack of access to good medical care dissuades retirees from wealthier countries, such as the United States and the United Kingdom, from retiring in the Caribbean. These retirees represent a lost potential source of income for the region.[5]

Working with the Barbados government on its HIV/AIDS programs, I saw firsthand the effects of the loss of healthcare workers to the United States has on even a relatively well-off country.

The exodus has included highly skilled public-health workers as well as clinicians. The Ministry of Health itself suffered an extreme shortage of monitoring and evaluation (M&E) experts. M&E experts are vital to an effective healthcare system because they use their knowledge in mathematics, research, and public health to collect and analyze data from healthcare programs to improve their management, provide accountability, and plan for the future. The widespread emigration had left just one M&E specialist available for the HIV/AIDS program. She herself was taking advantage of the shortage and gaming the system by regularly threatening to leave and work overseas, creating constant instability in the program.

In addition to my stint in Barbados, as I encountered country after country in which the fundamental problem was the shortage of healthcare workers, I was surprised to find that no significant World Bank grants or loans were addressing that problem. Finally I found a consultant, tucked away in a corner of the World Bank, who was studying this issue. Dr. Demissie Habte was the former dean of the Addis Ababa University, Faculty of Medicine, in Ethiopia, and the former director of the renowned International Centre for Diarrheal Disease Research, in Bangladesh. Drawing on his experience as both medical-school dean and manager of a large healthcare system, he was developing approaches to address the healthcare-worker shortage in developing countries. Together we wrote the first draft of a proposal for a World Bank program that would work on solutions to the global health-workforce crisis.

That work eventually led to the World Bank's African Health Workforce Program, which I coordinated, to assist countries in making better use of their healthcare workers and in training more. But these countries struggle to train more workers and help the existing workers to be more productive in the face of the constant loss of their best staff. It's like trying to build a house on an unstable foundation. At the same time, instead of training sufficient numbers of healthcare workers, rich countries are importing them from poor countries. With what I had seen as a clinician and learned as a global health-policy expert, it wasn't difficult to see how the two problems were linked.

Yet the connection between the two crises was completely off the radar in the American domestic-healthcare debate and among the global-health community. One reason the issue was receiving so little attention was ignorance; the US domestic health field and the global health field are large and complex areas of study, and no one expert can be expected to understand the whole field. But there is another explanation for the fact that no one addressed the linkages between the two healthcare-worker crises: The United States is the largest funder both of the World Health Organization and of global health aid in general, and no one wanted to be seen as biting the hand that fed them. No one wanted to be seen as blaming the United States for exacerbating the healthcare-worker shortage in developing countries, or, for that matter, for not effectively addressing the same issue at home.

The issues are complex and require complex analysis and solutions. But promising steps, at least in my experience, can come in surprising ways.

In addition to my work in global health, I've always kept active in US domestic health-policy work, figuring that my experience in the healthcare systems of dozens of different countries could contribute a fresh perspective to this country's healthcare challenges. Most recently, that work has been through Hope Street Group, a bipartisan volunteer organization that promotes economic opportunity. The Hope Street Group works with elected leaders from both parties, as well as with many kinds of experts, to develop business-friendly solutions to our greatest economic and social challenges, including education, employment, and access to healthcare. From the Hope Street Group's perspective, poor health and lack of access to healthcare are a serious economic problem. Sick workers cannot contribute to the economy, and large numbers of people with preventable disability drag the economy down. The maladaptive approach to solving our healthcare-workforce shortage by bringing in healthcare workers from abroad interested the Hope Street Group because it is an obvious loss of opportunity for Americans who seek careers in healthcare.

In partnership with health-insurance companies, large corporations, and assorted healthcare companies, the Hope Street Group is working to bring potential solutions to the US health-workforce shortage and maldistribution to the attention of elected leaders and to implement the most promising ideas. The main challenge is not so much the lack of good technical solutions to this crisis as the lack of solutions acceptable to all the important stakeholders. Many such solutions are outlined in this book. Our work is going forward and remains a bright spot of hope.

The production and distribution of healthcare workers is no Washington parlor game. The decisions we make about who we train to be health workers, how we train them, how many we train, and where we incentivize them to work directly affects the lives of millions of people, here and abroad. I urge you to think about that the next time you talk to your political representatives or healthcare leaders.

Dr. Kate Tulenko
Alexandria, Virginia
June 2011

Notes

1 "Locum Tenens Industry Fact Sheet," LocumTenens.com, accessed June 6, 2010, at www.locumtenens.com/lt/media/gallery/pdf/LocumTenens-Industry.pdf.

2 UNAIDS, *Global Report: UNAIDS Report on the Global AIDS Epidemic 2010* (Geneva: WHO, 2010), 202.

3 "HIV and AIDS in the Caribbean," AVERT, accessed June 19, 2009, at www.avert.org/aids-caribbean.htm.

4 "Caribbean Growth Hurt by Nursing Shortage," Reuters, accessed July 18, 2010, at www.reuters.com/article/2010/03/02/nurses-caribbean-idUSN0250417020100302.

5 World Bank, *The Nurse Labour and Education Markets in the English-Speaking CARICOM: Issues and Options for Reform* (Washington, DC: World Bank, 2009).

Acknowledgments

I would like to thank Dr. Tim Baker for all his support. It's amazing what you can do when someone believes in you.

Thanks to my agent, Andy Ross, and to Phyllis Deutsch at the University Press of New England for helping make the book a reality.

There are too many other people to thank personally. Thanks to all of you who gave interviews, offered encouragement and advice, and gave feedback on chapters. Not only did you make this book possible; you also kept it from being a lonely endeavor.

The views and opinions expressed in this book are those of Dr. Tulenko alone and do not necessarily represent those of her employers or funders.

INSOURCED

Introduction

Approximately 15 percent of all healthcare workers and 25 percent of all physicians in the United States were born and educated elsewhere.[1] This means that 1.5 million healthcare jobs are "insourced," occupied by foreign-born, foreign-trained workers brought into the United States on special visas earmarked for healthcare jobs. This number is 50 percent greater than the total number of jobs in the US auto-manufacturing industry. It's amazing to consider that in 2008 and 2009, the auto industry, which makes up just 3.6 percent of the US economy, received a $97 billion bailout. If we estimate that each of these 1.5 million insourced healthcare jobs has an average wage of $60,000, that's $90 billion a year in wages going to people brought into the United States to work rather than training Americans to do the same jobs.

The healthcare industry makes up 16 percent of our economy. Yet even in these days of close to 9 percent unemployment, we do not invest enough money in our young people to train them for jobs in healthcare—an already understaffed industry that will have to serve an additional 32 million people once the provisions of the 2010 health-reform law take full effect. Instead, when faced with pressure from hospitals and nursing homes for more healthcare workers, the federal government grants visas to import nurses, physicians, pharmacists, physical therapists, and many other types of healthcare workers from countries that can ill afford to lose them.

In some US industries, the outcome of globalization is positive or neutral. Take the sugar industry. Due to lower labor and land costs and better weather conditions, it's far cheaper to grow sugar cane in the Caribbean than sugar beets in North Dakota. As import taxes fall, global transportation improves, and the number of sugar beet farms in the United States declines, more Americans are sweetening their cereal with sugar from Jamaican sugar cane. Americans save money buying cheaper sugar; the economy of the poorer sugar-growing countries improves, lifting thousands of people out of poverty; and the few displaced American sugar beet farmers generally find other work. But sugar is not a strategic commodity. If CARICOM, the Caribbean Community, were to halt sugar exports to the United States, we would experience no crisis. Sugar is not essential to our diet or life, and we have plenty of substitutes, from honey and corn syrup to NutraSweet. If necessary, within a year we could again be producing sugar in the United States.

The US healthcare industry is 200 times larger than the US tire-manufacturing industry, yet President Obama risked a trade war with China, our biggest trade partner, over tires.[2] He was understandably trying to protect well-paying manufacturing jobs for American workers. Yet each year, we bring thousands of nurses from China to work in even better-paying jobs, rather than train young people in this country to become nurses. The irony is that the economic costs of "insourcing" healthcare workers, including the loss of jobs no longer available to Americans, are far greater than the costs when we import Chinese tires. In 2003 the Commission on Graduates of Foreign Nursing Schools (CGFNS), a US-based nongovernmental organization that administers the US nursing licensing exam to foreign-trained nurses, opened a testing center in Beijing. The opening of this center initiated a "mushrooming" of new nursing schools in China and led to credible predictions that China will soon become the number one source of foreign-trained nurses imported to the United States.[3]

Given the publicity and furor over the loss of manufacturing jobs, the lack of protest over healthcare-worker insourcing is surprising. Congress passed legislation and President George W. Bush signed a law in 2007 to protect the American sock industry from the rival Honduran sock industry.[4] Yes, that's right: socks. Protecting a few hundred $15-an-hour sock-manufacturing jobs based *solely* in the small town of Fort Payne, Alabama, was worth acting on. Yet insourcing hundreds of thousands of $60-an-hour healthcare jobs has prompted no such similarly high-level response from our leaders.

Instead, on a regular basis, Congress approves and presidents from both political parties sign legislation to enable the legal entry of an ever-increasing number of foreign healthcare workers. Each year, about 20,000 new healthcare-specific visas are issued for these workers.[5]

The United States has traditionally not allowed strategic industries to be outsourced. That's why the US steel industry and the US car industry have received bailout after bailout. Access to enough steel and automobiles is essential to our economy; without a sufficient supply of each, our economy would be severely damaged. It's time we acknowledged that the health of the population is just as important as steel and autos in keeping our economy strong. Healthcare is too important to risk continuing to insource it.

It's not just a matter of protecting and expanding jobs for American workers. Every year, thousands of Americans die, and the health of thousands more is compromised, because of the shortage of healthcare workers in every one of the healthcare professions.[6]

On the surface, insourcing may appear to be a harmless or even win-win solution to the country's healthcare-worker shortage. The hospital receives a much-needed worker, and the worker escapes life in a struggling country for a better life here. But we should be training more people in this country to work in those professions, especially people from rural poor and minority communities. Rather than investing in our own people and communities, however, we have decided to take the best and brightest workers from struggling countries.[7]

Many foreign-trained healthcare workers, no matter how smart, are not adequately prepared for practice in the fast-paced, high-tech world of US medicine.[8] Whether in operating rooms, hospital wards, or nursing homes, inadequately qualified and poorly oriented foreign healthcare workers endanger the lives of their patients, as well as the lives and careers of their American-trained colleagues.

But the main reason for this country's rise in unnecessary deaths and delayed care is understaffing—a result of the failure to train and place enough healthcare workers, especially in rural and underserved communities. Americans who live in rural areas make fewer visits to healthcare providers and are less likely to receive preventive care.[9] The infant-mortality rate for African Americans is twice that for the average American;[10] Latinos are twice as likely as white Americans to die from diabetes. These health disparities are due in large part to a lack of healthcare workers, especially primary-care workers, in their communities. The quick fix has been importing foreign healthcare workers for these unfilled positions. Unfortunately, once these workers fulfill their initial contracts, most move to communities without healthcare-worker shortages; in fact, foreign-trained healthcare workers are more likely to practice in the well-served, major metropolitan areas than their American-trained counterparts.

Even if good foreign-trained healthcare workers were here in numbers adequate to meet our needs, the US healthcare system is about encounter a tidal wave of demand as 78 million baby boomers approach their sixties. Older people make, on average, six visits to a healthcare provider a year, compared with two visits per year for people under 60. The healthcare workforce is aging, too: More than 50 percent of practicing healthcare workers are eligible to retire during the next 10 years, which will leave us with fewer workers to treat more and sicker patients.

In the eyes of healthcare employers, of course, insourcing healthcare workers appears to offer many benefits. Most doctors and nurses in developing countries earn a fraction of what American doctors and nurses earn: A Caribbean nurse makes around $1,000 a month; an Ethiopian physician, about $100 a month. Not only are foreign-trained healthcare workers accustomed to lower salaries and quality of life, but they also carry little or no education debt, while their American-trained colleagues typically graduate with five- and six-figure debt burdens. With average student debt burdens of $155,000[11] for newly graduated physicians and $30,375 for nurses,[12] American-trained health workers require a higher salary just to help pay for their education. Trained in a much more hierarchical environment, foreign workers are much less likely to unionize, or even express dissatisfaction with their work. As the percentage of imported healthcare workers increases, their attitudes toward salary and terms of employment undermine the bargaining power of US workers, and even affect the important feedback loop between employees and management.

Polls indicate that 70 to 80 percent of Americans want to reduce the rate of immigration into the United States.[13] Yet the American public is not aware of our policy of using healthcare-worker-specific visas to solve the healthcare-worker shortage.

Some legislators who publicly support stabilizing immigration consistently vote to increase the number of healthcare-worker-specific visas granted each year.

It's not that American citizens don't want to become healthcare workers and fill these jobs. This distinction is critical, because every industry that has brought in foreign workers has argued that American workers won't do the work for the prevailing wage, or won't do the work no matter how high the pay is. In the healthcare industry, this argument does not apply. US citizens want the jobs. They just can't access the training. The United States does not have enough positions in health-professional schools to meet industry demands.

The tens of thousands of qualified nursing school and medical school applicants who are denied entry to school each year permanently lose out on their chosen careers, work that is consistently ranked in the top tier of salaries, with excellent benefits and almost guaranteed job security. This loss of career opportunity is even greater for rural and minority young people, who are grossly underrepresented in the higher-level health professions, such as physicians and nurses, and overrepresented in the lower-level professions, such as technicians and home health assistants. Something is wrong when so many young Americans are forced to pursue other, lower-paying careers at a time when we desperately need *more* healthcare providers. In exchange we get foreign healthcare workers who are less well trained (they consistently score lower on licensing exams than US-trained healthcare workers) and far less culturally competent than native-born Americans.

The most tragic and most preventable effect of our hiring so many healthcare workers from other countries is the unnecessary deaths of hundreds of thousands of men, women, and children in developing countries. The World Health Organization (WHO) estimates that each year more than 10 million people die needlessly, from easily treatable maladies such as diarrhea, pneumonia, malaria, tuberculosis, vaccine-preventable diseases, and complications of childbirth. The WHO Global Health Workforce Alliance estimates that there are a billion people alive today who will never see a health worker in their lives. In Ethiopia, one in 10 Ethiopian children will die before his or her fifth birthday—yet there are more Ethiopian physicians in the Chicago area than in all of Ethiopia, which, with 80 million people, is the second most populous country in Africa. As their most skilled nurses emigrate to work in US nursing homes, middle-income countries such as Jamaica and Trinidad have nurse-vacancy rates of 60 percent or higher.

Throughout the developing world, nurses, pharmacists, physical therapists, and many other types of healthcare workers are being approached and offered 10 times their salaries to practice in modern US healthcare facilities with state-of-the-art technologies. Even the most dedicated, socially conscious worker would be tempted by such an offer. A colleague of mine relayed a conversation he'd had with the head of the Nursing Council of Kenya, who told him about the damage the exodus of senior nurses was doing to her country's healthcare system. In the next breath, she confessed that the next time he visited Kenya, she might not be there. She was thinking about emigrating herself.

Our unofficial policy of relying on the world's poorest countries to pay for the training of workers whom we then entice and bring to this country is devastating healthcare systems around the world. The loss to a developing country when a single physician, representing what may be a significant portion of their total number of physicians, emigrates is far greater than our gain. Our failure to provide education for our own citizens and to better plan for healthcare staffing and distribution does not justify hiring nurses and physicians from the countries that can least afford to lose them. How many additional deaths, how much more needless disability and suffering, will we allow this misguided policy to cause?

And consider American competitiveness. Certain industries are vital to US global leadership. Recognizing their importance, we protect those industries. We don't allow them to move overseas and make the United States vulnerable to the actions of other countries. Poor farmers in the developing world can certainly grow food staples more cheaply than American farmers do. But because of the strategic importance of the US food supply, we subsidize some basic food crops, such as corn and soybeans.

And yet we are overreliant on foreign healthcare workers to meet our most basic health needs. This is particularly dangerous because many countries, almost completely drained of healthcare workers and tired of subsidizing the US healthcare system, are trying to slam the door shut for emigrating healthcare workers. Meantime, of the world's wealthiest nations, the United States has the worst health outcomes, with lower life expectancies and higher rates of deaths from preventable causes. In infant mortality, for instance, we rank 27th, behind Poland and Hungary. Our disability levels are higher than in most former-Soviet countries.[14]

If the United States is to remain competitive in the global economy, we need a *healthy workforce*. In order to achieve that, we need a *healthcare workforce* made up of adequate numbers of properly trained physicians, nurses, pharmacists, community-health workers, and other healthcare providers.

By picking up this book, you have started on a journey from the hallowed halls of academic medicine to Capitol Hill, from small-town, rural America to big healthcare corporations, from international recruiting agencies to myriad developing nations. We'll explore the extent of the healthcare-worker deficit in the United States and how it is going to worsen, very soon. We'll investigate a healthcare-worker education system with incentives that drive education costs up rather than lowering them, and that trains workers to seek higher salaries and ivory towers rather than to meet the country's real health needs. We'll see an education-funding system that does not recognize the true cost of education and for which there is no accountability to the communities they are supposed to serve. We will learn how the United States fell into a system that depends on importing healthcare workers, and how Congress has increasingly supported that dependence.

We will look into the abuses of the international recruiting industry and see how foreign doctors and nurses arrive here with little or no understanding of American medicine or of the needs and expectations of American patients. We'll see what happens to the patients, communities, and healthcare systems when their healthcare workers emigrate. We'll consider international attempts to solve this problem, some of them more successful than others. And finally, we will develop sustainable alternatives to the mass insourcing of healthcare workers.

Grab your passport and let's begin!

1

Shortage in the Land of Abundance

Every year, as the United States imports more than 20,000 foreign-trained workers on special visas earmarked for the healthcare sector, American nursing and medical schools turn away tens of thousands of qualified applicants. These Americans are forever denied a career in one of the country's most economically rewarding fields. Even more troubling, the gap between the supply of and demand for healthcare workers continues to grow—a literally life-and-death problem. Why is it happening?

With more than 308 million people, the United States is the world's third most populous country, behind China and India. Health is this country's largest and fastest-growing industry: More than 16 percent of all the money spent by consumers and the government goes to healthcare. By 2017, we will spend 19.5 percent—almost 20 percent!—of our Gross Domestic Product on healthcare.[1] If you want figures, $2.5 trillion—that's with a *t*—was spent on the US healthcare industry in 2009, up from $2.3 trillion the previous year.[2]

Yet we have a huge deficit in the number of people needed to run this industry—we do not have enough doctors, nurses, pharmacists, and other healthcare workers to protect the health of all our people. Worse still, the shortages are most severe among the most highly trained and highly paid healthcare workers, such as doctors and nurses, who provide the majority of direct, hands-on care. These are the very areas in which we import the most workers from other countries. Yet the gap between supply and demand is growing larger each day.

For the patients, this causes more than frustration and inconvenience. It means something far worse than longer waits for an appointment with your doctor, or having to drive farther because the physicians or hospitals nearest your home are not taking new patients. Unable to be seen by a physician in a timely manner, many people either delay care or do not seek care at all, which can lead to the escalation of easily treatable conditions, such as simple infections or early diabetes, and much higher rates of permanent disability and death. More directly and dramatically, nurses and physicians trying to care for too many patients in clinics and hospitals are more likely to make medical errors or overlook medical conditions that can result in disability or death.

Pushing the "call" button on a hospital bed and wondering when a nurse will arrive is so common it has achieved the status of a joke, although there is nothing funny about being in pain. Every family has a loved one who has waited for what seemed an eternity to receive pain medication, who has felt extreme anxiety while waiting for someone to explain why an alarm went off in the room, or who has suffered the indignity of soiling him- or herself while waiting for a nurse to bring a bedpan or help the patient into the bathroom.

But there are far more tragic stories caused by the healthcare-worker shortage. In one case, a woman bled to death in a Los Angeles emergency room while vomiting blood, as she pleaded to be seen by a doctor.[3] In another, a woman bled to death following a routine hysterectomy, because there was only one registered nurse on the ward, and she was caring for 40 patients.[4]

With such inadequate staffing, it is impossible for a single registered nurse, no matter how qualified, to identify a patient in trouble and respond in a timely and effective manner. I could fill this whole book with heartbreaking stories like this.

The United States Institute of Medicine's landmark report on medical errors, "To Err Is Human," determined that each year, medical errors in American hospitals cause an estimated 100,000 people to die unnecessarily and injure an additional 1.5 million.[5] This was back in 1999. And the number one cause of medical error, even then? Mistakes made by nurses and physicians forced by staff shortages to work long shifts or to care for large numbers of patients.

A study published in the *Journal of the American Medical Association* in 2002 found that nurses with high patient loads reported greater job dissatisfaction and emotional distress and that "failure to retain nurses contributes to avoidable patient deaths."[6] A few years later, the Joint Commission on Accreditation of Healthcare Organizations (JCAHO), an independent, not-for-profit organization that accredits more than 17,000 healthcare organizations in the United States, looked into the damage caused by the nursing shortage. In its report, issued in 2009, the commission concluded that this shortage results in tens of thousands of injuries, prolonged hospitalizations, and deaths in both hospitals and nursing homes.[7] The report found that due to the healthcare-worker shortage, responses to catastrophic events such as natural disasters or terrorist attacks, and even primary care, are compromised.

In another study published in the *Journal of the American Medical Association* in 2002, University of Pennsylvania researchers found that patients had a greater chance of dying after surgery when there were too few nurses—the fewer the nurses, the greater the chance. The Associated Press reported that "each additional patient in a nurse's workload translated to about a 7 percent increase in the likelihood the patient would die within 30 days of admission. For example, the difference between four and six patients per nurse translated to a 14 percent increase in mortality, while the difference between four and eight patients increased the likelihood of dying by 31 percent."[8]

Just a 10 percent reduction in registered nurses per patient has been linked to a 14 percent increase in medical errors.[9] According to a study conducted by the Harvard School of Public Health and published in the *New England Journal of Medicine* in 2002, 53 percent of doctors cite the nursing shortage as the number one cause of medical errors.[10] In hospitals and clinics, nurses directly administer most of the drugs, and an overworked nurse can easily administer a drug improperly (wrong dose, wrong drug, wrong patient) or fail to catch an error in a physician's order.

Overburdened healthcare workers have less time to assess each patient for complications, and less time to communicate with other healthcare workers regarding their patients. This information exchange is especially critical at "sign-out," when doctors and nurses going off duty apprise the new shift of the patients' medical needs. A doctor or nurse who does not get an adequate sign-out on a patient is less able to anticipate and address his or her problems. The more patients a doctor or nurse has to sign out, the higher the chance that the communication will not be adequate.

Further compounding the challenge is the fact that the average annual turnover rate among nurses is 14 percent.[11] This means that at any given hospital or clinic, 14 percent of the nurses working there today will have accepted a job elsewhere a year from now. The high turnover is driven by a salary and benefit bidding war as healthcare facilities compete over the limited supply of nurses.

Such turnover threatens patient health, because a large portion of the staff is less familiar with the patient population, the health facility, the procedures in case of a patient emergency, and the location of emergency equipment. How does the hospital announce an emergency code? Where's the code cart with the emergency supplies? If the patient cannot breathe on her own, where on the cart are the intubation supplies? As a physician who frequently works in hospitals and clinics with which I am unfamiliar, I can tell you that my ability to respond is diminished when I don't know a facility well.

Also in 2002, the Center for Medicare and Medicaid Services found that 90 percent of all long-term nursing homes lack the minimum nurse staffing to deliver even the most basic care.[12] Understaffing of nurses has caused both medical and nursing-home facilities to face legal charges of negligence. Since state law is usually quite clear on nurse-staffing requirements, there is normally no recourse for hospitals or nursing homes but to plead no contest to the charges.

A prime example is that of Pleasant Care Corporation, the second-largest nursing-home chain in California, which did not hire enough staff to provide each resident with at least three hours of nursing care for every 24 hours they were in the facility. After the state attorney general filed criminal and negligence charges against the company, it settled a multimillion-dollar lawsuit in 2006 by paying $1.35 million in civil penalties and reimbursing the state for its investigation into its facilities.

According to the *Napa Valley Register* (one of the nursing homes was in Napa), "prosecutors estimate the company will pay more than $2 million alone to hire enough nursing staff to meet a quota of 3.2 hours spent per day with each nursing home resident." It's quite likely the company has had to hire foreign nurses.

You might think such understaffing is due to efforts to cut costs or raise profits, but that is not usually the case. Many hospitals lose money if they don't have enough nurses and have to turn away paying patients. Every day, thousands of advertised, budgeted-for nursing jobs go unfilled. During just one month at the end of 2010, one nursing job site, www.NursingJobs.org, had 1,000 nursing jobs posted. In 2009, when the JCAHO nursing shortage report was written, there were 126,000 budgeted-for but unfilled nursing positions in the United States.

The staff-shortage problem has become so grave that nurses have begun going on strike over the dangerously low nurse-to-patient ratios. This concern over staffing ratios was the root cause of the country's largest-ever nursing strike, which occurred when 12,000 nurses walked out of hospitals, nursing homes, and clinics in Minneapolis and St. Paul, Minnesota, in 2010.[13]

Even if we could import enough foreign-trained healthcare workers to fill every vacancy in every hospital, nursing home, and clinic, the medical errors, large and small, would continue. All across the country, medical errors due to cultural clashes are on the rise, too. Most foreign healthcare workers are unfamiliar with and untrained in the subtleties of this country's varied cultures. Likewise, many American patients have little or no understanding of the cultures of their foreign caregivers. Differing attitudes of patient and caregiver toward health, illness, medications, death, and dying—even toward gays and lesbians, domestic violence, and abortion—can negatively affect a patient's health.

For example, in some countries, infants born with conditions known to be fatal within a few days or weeks are not considered "live births" and are not recorded in birth registries. You can imagine how this attitude might affect the care given these infants during their brief lives. In many countries, homosexuality is illegal; in some, it is a capital offense. You can understand how practitioners trained in these countries would have a different attitude toward screening for homosexuality in teens—which is important, to address the social-stigma issues and the higher suicide rates in this teen population—as well as toward patients who identify themselves as gay. Similarly, in some countries, fatal diagnoses are often not communicated to patients, only to the patient's closest relative or relatives. Needless to say, this approach clashes with American ideals of self-determination and the right to know about one's own health.

An Indonesian physician colleague of mine once sadly told me about her worst "missed case." Indonesia is a Muslim country, with strict social norms regarding sex outside of marriage. My colleague was caring for a young woman complaining of abdominal pain. Because the woman was not married, the physician did not consider possible reproductive-tract causes, such as pregnancy or sexually transmitted disease. And because of the social stigma, the woman did not communicate her sexual history to the doctor. My colleague diagnosed the problem as a relatively mild gastrointestinal disorder. Later, the woman died of complications from an abortion. An American-trained physician would have automatically considered reproductive-health issues as a cause of abdominal pain in a woman, no matter what the patient told her. American-trained physicians are taught that when patients are asked for their medical history, sexual history is the most frequently undisclosed part.

Language barriers obviously affect quality of care. Until recently, foreign-trained nurses and physicians had to pass the Test of English as a Foreign Language (TOEFL). The argument for dropping the TOEFL requirement is that all healthcare workers have to pass clinical exams in English and the TOEFL is therefore redundant. But there is a huge difference between passing a clinical exam in English and passing the more rigorous TOEFL. Only the TOEFL could guarantee that the health workers will be able to communicate effectively with their patients, especially on socially sensitive issues and on matters of life and death. When I asked the owner of a major international nurse-recruitment agency the biggest challenge her nurses faced in working in this country, she said one of the main problems was understanding American accents, particularly those of less educated patients — a group that already has poor access to care.

Large numbers of foreign nurses work in nursing homes, where language barriers are a particular concern. Because of a general lack of contact with nonnative English speakers, seniors have more trouble than younger people understanding foreign accents; seniors also have the hearing and language-comprehension difficulties that come with advancing age. Many seniors with dementia or Parkinson's disease also have difficulty articulating their words or forming their sentences, making them more difficult to understand. This difficulty that seniors have communicating with foreign-trained workers not only affects their health care but can also compound their feelings of social isolation.

"Physicians bury their mistakes," and no one hears this more than funeral directors. In talking with funeral directors I was surprised to hear the number of complaints they receive and lawsuits they were aware of from family members of people who had died while being cared for by foreign physicians. Stephen Kemp, a funeral director, former professor at Wayne State University School of Mortuary Science and former president of the Michigan Funeral Directors Association, told me example after example of families who felt that they had not been able to communicate with their family member's doctors. Many of the patients were cared for in the St. John's Health System Hospitals in Detroit, where most of the intensive care physicians are from the

Middle East. According to Kemp, the most common complaint is that the family was never properly told what was wrong with their loved one. In addition, families report that foreign-trained physicians are less likely to talk to women family members and are more resistant to answering family members' questions than American doctors. From his experience, foreign-trained doctors need better listening skills, better communications skills, and cultural and sensitivity training.

If known flaws in the American auto industry caused as many accidents and deaths as the American healthcare industry, there would be a tremendous uproar. In 2010, the defective gas pedals that led to the recall of hundreds of thousands of Toyota vehicles (and cost more than $2 billion) caused 34 deaths. I've heard of people who are afraid to buy Toyotas now and are switching to other automakers. Why are we unafraid, then, of walking into our own clinics, emergency rooms, and hospitals, where tens of thousands of people die unnecessarily each year?

Aging Doctors, Aging Patients

Just as in so many other facets of our society, baby boomers—those Americans born between 1946 and 1964—are set to put enormous pressure on our healthcare system. The oldest are just turning 66, entering the period of life in which they will consume more medical care than they did during the entire previous 65 years.

People 60 and older make an average of six visits to a doctor per year, compared with two visits per year for people under 60. Seniors have higher rates of heart disease, cancer, diabetes, stroke, dementia, and other long-term, debilitating diseases, requiring far more contact with the healthcare system. This need spans all the components of the system and the healthcare workers who keep the system functioning: in-home care, clinic-based care, hospital care, and long-term-facility care.

The increased demand with age for healthcare services is even greater when you look at hospitalization rates. Americans under the age of 15 account for less than 7 percent of all hospitalizations; those aged 15 to 44 account for 31 percent; those aged 45 to 64, for 25 percent. Americans 65 and older account for 38 percent of all hospitalizations—more than one-third, even though this age group is only 12 percent of the population. At 70 million strong, the boomers' combined need for more healthcare will result in a significantly increased demand for healthcare workers.

At the same time that this increase in demand will happen, baby boomer doctors and nurses will be retiring, which means we'll have fewer healthcare workers just as the country has begun needing more. According to the Department of Labor, 817,000 physicians are currently active in the United States.[14] Over one-third of them are more than 50 years old. Merritt Hawkins & Associates, a physician-placement firm, published a worrisome study focused on physicians 50 to 65 years old. They studied this age group because, comprising 38 percent of all practicing physicians, it is the largest cohort of physicians in the United States. Only 28 percent of these physicians reported that they plan to be practicing full time in 2013. In three years, 38 percent plan to retire completely; 28 percent plan to substantially reduce their workload; and 10 percent said they plan to switch to nonclinical work, such as hospital management or insurance-industry work.[15]

Looking ahead less than 10 years, the Association of American Medical Colleges (AAMC) estimates that 250,000 active physicians in the 50-and-over age group will retire by 2020.[16]

Meanwhile, we don't even have a physician-to-population ratio equal to that of other developed countries. Our current physician-to-population ratio is 2.4 per 1,000, and it is expected to fall over the next decade. The average physician-to-population ratio in developed countries is three practicing physicians per 1,000 people. In that regard, the United States ranks 23rd, behind Greece, Spain, the Czech Republic, the Slovak Republic, and Hungary.[17] In addition to a lower physician-to-population ratio, the United States has worse health outcomes than most of these countries.

The shortage of healthcare workers is already so acute that the Department of Health and Human Services' Bureau of Health Professions has created a category called Health Professional Shortage Area (HPSA): a geographical area with less than one primary-care provider (physician, nurse practitioner, or physician assistant) per 2,000 people. The 6,000-plus HPSAs have 65 million people living in them, in all states and in both rural and urban communities. There are also more than 4,000 dental HPSAs, with 49 million people, and more than 3,000 mental-health HPSAs, with 80 million people.

Estimates of the coming shortage of physicians vary, but most experts agree that by 2020 the United States will need 125,000 new physicians *just to fill vacancies*. Should the United States decide to increase its physician-to-population ratio to equal that of other developed countries, by 2020 we will have a shortage of 500,000 physicians.[18]

And the shortage is not limited to primary-care physicians. Most specialists are in short supply as well. During the past 25 years, the overall number of general surgeons per 100,000 people has declined by 26 percent.[19] As the population ages, the ratio of specialists whose services are demanded primarily by seniors—urologists, say, to choose one example—will decline. This will happen as the number of seniors in this country grows by 36 percent.[20]

Given these numbers, the Association of American Medical Colleges (AAMC) has recommended a 30 percent increase in the number of physicians graduating from medical school each year, as well as an increase in the number of residencies, the next step for med school graduates. Such a scale-up is possible, but it will be difficult if, as the next chapter shows, our medical schools continue to focus mainly on research rather than on what should be their primary mission: training physicians.

Even if the United States had the appropriate number of physicians to meet our needs, the ratio of primary-care physicians to specialists is out of balance. Primary-care physicians—whether family practitioners, general internal-medicine practitioners, or general pediatricians—provide the bulk of care in this country. In addition to the direct care they provide, they coordinate their patients' care with specialists and are the one provider familiar with the whole care of their patients. But today, only about 22 percent of newly graduated doctors go into primary care, and the number is declining year by year.[21] To provide the proper ratio between primary-care and specialty practitioners, more than 50 percent of medical students should enter primary-care residencies.

Exacerbating the problem is the fact that today's doctors are working fewer hours per week than in the past. According to a 2010 study published in the *Journal of the American Medical Association*, the average workweek for nonresident physicians declined by 7.1 percent between 1996 and 2008, from 55 to 51 hours per week.[22]

Resident physicians—new medical school graduates receiving in-depth training in their specialty area—have had little control over the number of hours they work, but it has clearly been too many. In 2003, the Accreditation Council for Graduate Medical Education instituted new work-limit regulations to protect the health and safety of residents and the patients they care for. These regulations call for residents to work no more than 80 hours per week, with a minimum of 10 hours between shifts and at least one 24-hour period off each week.

Some may believe the reason doctors are working fewer hours is that more than half of the new physicians since 2005 are women. But an equally strong "feminization" has occurred in the field of law, and to some extent in engineering, while the hours worked in those fields has remained stable over the last 30 years. Although women physicians do tend to work fewer hours than their male counterparts, young male physicians are working fewer hours than older male physicians.

This trend may be attributable to the fact that top-of-the-class men and women seeking both a rewarding career (intellectually, socially, and financially) and a good work-life balance are choosing to go into the field of medicine because it does not require the 80-hour workweeks of their high-achieving classmates in legal, finance, and corporate careers. Whatever the reason for this phenomenon, a decrease of 5.7 percent in working hours per week is equivalent to a loss of 36,000 physicians from the active workforce. As the older physicians—the ones who work longer hours—retire, this trend will no doubt continue, and the United States will experience an even greater decrease in active physicians.

Nurses Are Aging, Too

Nurses make up the largest segment of the US healthcare workforce. According to the Department of Health and Human Services and the American Nursing Association, the United States has more than 2.8 million working registered nurses, or RNs.[23] That number is greater than the populations of 38 countries, including Latvia, Slovenia, and Namibia, and is roughly three times the number of physicians currently working in this country. Yet it is greatly insufficient to meet our basic healthcare needs.

The number of registered nurses graduating from nursing schools in the United States has leveled off at around 71,000 per year.[24] And, just as with physicians, a wave of retirements will soon erode the numbers of working nurses. The average age of American registered nurses has been increasing since the statistic was first tracked, in 1980. Only 8 percent of RNs are under 30 years old, down from 25 percent in 1980. This number looks even worse when you consider that the average age of working nurses is 47, and that 41 percent of all US RNs are older than 50—up from 25 percent in 1980 and 33 percent in 2000.[25] Clearly, a large percentage of nurses—particularly the senior nurses, who hold critical positions in hospitals—are baby boomers on the cusp on retirement. In a survey conducted in 2006, the Bernard Hodes Group, a human-resources firm, found that 55 percent of senior nurses are planning to retire by 2020.[26]

And, just as with physicians, we don't have enough nurses at work *now*. Three-quarters of all advertised hospital vacancies are for nurses. According to the American Hospital Association, 116,000 nurses are needed right now to fill open, advertised positions in hospitals and clinics. Another 19,400 advertised positions are available in nursing homes.

Those vacancies are just the positions that hospital and nursing-home administrators are looking to fill. Some experts estimate that an *additional 100,000 nurses are needed immediately* to bring all nursing homes into compliance with state nurse-to-patient ratios. Peter Buerhaus, chairman of the National Health Workforce Commission and director of the Center for Interdisciplinary Health Workforce Studies at Vanderbilt University School of Nursing, in Nashville, Tennessee, noted that while the current recession has caused massive layoffs in many fields, the hiring of nurses has continued—and that the shortage of registered nurses will balloon to 260,000 in the next few years.[27] The predicted nursing shortage will be twice as severe as any non-war-related labor shortage the United States has ever experienced, in any sector.

But even this estimate—a shortfall of more than a quarter-million nurses—may be too low. The Health Resources and Services Administration (HRSA), the government office responsible for increasing access to healthcare for those who are underserved, has predicted that by 2020 the United States will be short more than *1 million nurses*.[28] This will represent a greater than 20 percent deficit in the number of nurses needed to provide healthcare to Americans—a nurse-vacancy rate more in line with those in developing and postconflict countries, such as Zambia and Malawi, than with those in other wealthy countries.

Since we are not educating enough nurses to replace those who are retiring,[29] we certainly won't be able to meet the increased demands of the aging population. According to the Council on Physician and Nurse Supply, an independent group of healthcare leaders, an additional 30,000 nurses must graduate from US nursing schools each year to meet our current and future healthcare needs. This would be a 30 percent increase in the number of new nurses each year.[30]

Pharmacists, Public-Health Workers, and Other Healthcare Providers

Nurses and physicians are the most prominent workers in our healthcare system, but across the United States, there are critical shortages of pharmacists, podiatrists, occupational therapists, physical therapists, audiologists, nutritionists, speech therapists, respiratory therapists, radiology technicians, and many other types of healthcare professionals. These healthcare workers function as part of a team supporting the care of the whole patient. As with any team, when one member is absent, it affects the work of all the others.

The most studied of these other workers are pharmacists, the third most common healthcare worker in our healthcare system after nurses and doctors. We have only half the pharmacists we need right now; according to the Association of Colleges of Pharmacy, another 150,000 will be required by 2020 to meet industry demand.[31] This is particularly worrisome because it takes eight years to train a pharmacist, and again, demand for the profession will only grow with the aging of the population. Older people use far more prescription drugs than younger people. According to the Kaiser Family Foundation, the average American age 18 or under has 4 prescriptions filled a year; the average 19- to 64-year-old has 11 prescriptions filled per year. The average American 65 years and older has 31 prescriptions filled each year.[32]

The huge deficit in American healthcare workers extends beyond clinical workers to those in the fields of public health and public safety: those healthcare workers for whom success means you aren't even aware that they are there. One week after the September 11 attacks, you may remember, deadly anthrax spores were sent to several media offices as well as to the offices of two US senators. The infected letters killed five people and severely sickened 17 others. Thousands of public-health workers were put on the case, both to protect the public's immediate health and to discover who was responsible for the poisonings.

Epidemiologists looked at those who were infected, trying to discover connections that might link them: a worksite, a political affiliation, a shared post office. Biochemists and molecular biologists worked to sequence the DNA of the anthrax spores to develop their molecular "fingerprint" and identify what laboratory or wild strain of anthrax they had come from. Infectious-disease experts recommended ways of protecting the public at large. Water engineers worked to protect, monitor, and treat our water supply. Public-health officers coordinated local responses. Public-health communications experts composed easy-to-understand messages to explain how to protect ourselves and to instill a level of concern high enough to provoke action but not high enough to cause panic.

These are the unsung heroes of our healthcare system. On a moment's notice, the "infectious-disease detectives" in the CDC's Epidemic Intelligence Service travel anywhere, at home or around the globe, to study an outbreak of a disease that could affect us, whether hanta virus in the American Southwest, diarrheal outbreaks on US cruise ships, SARS in China, Ebola in Angola, swine flu in Mexico, or hepatitis A from green onions eaten in a Pennsylvania restaurant.[33]

Think how much worse the salmonella event in the summer of 2010 would have been if public-health officers had not noticed a spike in salmonella reports, investigated, and noted that what the people affected had in common was that they had recently eaten eggs. In the end, 250 people were sickened and half a billion potentially contaminated eggs were removed from store shelves. In fact, one of the vulnerabilities identified in this investigation was that the US Food and Drug Administration did not have enough food-safety specialists to adequately inspect the country's egg farms.

My office is in downtown Washington, DC, just two blocks from the White House. On the roofs of many of the buildings I walk past every day are radiation monitors watched over by radiation-health experts. In our heightened state of security alert, these workers regularly monitor our air, food, and water supplies.

After 9/11 and the anthrax poisonings, the federal government and state governments invested billions of dollars in the long-neglected fields of public health and safety. Later, in response to global pandemics such as the outbreaks of SARS, avian flu, and swine flu, the US government created tens of thousands more public-health jobs. In 2003, the total number of federal, state, and local public-health workers reached a peak of 556,000. The number of public-health workers has been declining ever since, despite increases in the number of budgeted public-health positions and increases in health threats and the US population.

Thousands of these jobs go unfilled because we do not invest enough in training new public-health workers. In some states, the vacancy rate for public-health workers is up to 20 percent. These jobs would go to epidemiologists who trace disease outbreaks to their origins, laboratory technicians who help identify disease-causing agents, quarantine officers who protect our health at US borders, and environmental-health workers who ensure that our water is safe to drink and our air is safe to breathe. This category of healthcare worker, too, is aging. The average age of a public-health worker is about 47. In many jurisdictions, about 45 percent of the public-health workers are expected to retire in the next few years.

More Demands on a Dwindling Supply

So the numbers of physicians, registered nurses, pharmacists, laboratory technicians, public-health workers, and all other categories of healthcare professionals are insufficient today, and the need in all fields will be greater tomorrow. But an aging healthcare workforce and too few new workers being trained to augment and replace them is just part of the problem. Many other factors are increasing the need for more healthcare workers.

Experts who look at technology through an economic lens will tell you that technological advances—from the cotton gin to the iPad—tend to reduce the need for human labor, so that fewer workers can produce more at a cheaper cost. But the reverse is true in medicine, where technological advances generally create additional labor needs.[34] Medical technological advances drive the demand for healthcare workers.

Both my grandfather, who passed away in 1980, and my father, who is seventy-five, began to suffer from osteoarthritis in their sixties. All that my grandfather's primary-care doctor could do was to offer him painkillers and a cane. Forty years later, when my father developed the same symptoms, much more could be done, by a whole team of healthcare professionals. His primary-care physician prescribed nonsteroidal anti-inflammatory medications that didn't just mask the pain; they slowed down the degradation of his joints. When the condition naturally progressed further, my father was referred to an orthopedic surgeon and a physical therapist. The orthopedic surgeon gave him steroid injections and, eventually, two artificial knees and two artificial hips, one of which has already been replaced. He has had dozens of radiology studies performed on his joints, keeping a team of radiologists busy. Through hundreds of visits to the physical therapist, my once-athletic father learned to walk again and how to strengthen the muscles around his affected joints to protect them from the impact stress of walking. The physical therapist also helped him walk again after his five joint replacements, each of which required the care of an operating-room team and a hospital-recovery team.

The good news is that my father is much more mobile than his father was at the same age. The bad news on the health-workforce side is that my father has made literally dozens of visits a year to healthcare providers, versus the handful of times a year my grandfather visited his physician. And that's just for one medical condition, osteoarthritis. He's also had numerous stress tests and cardiac catheterizations and endoscopies that were developed or made available after my grandfather passed away and that increase the demand for health workers. At 75, my father is statistically at high risk for heart disease, diabetes, cancer, depression, and dementia—all conditions far more common in seniors, and for which few interventions existed 40 years ago but for which there are now multiple interventions, each requiring a team of healthcare workers. HealthSouth, the nation's largest provider of in-patient rehabilitative-healthcare services, reports that 72 percent of its patients are considered "medically complex," with six or more diagnoses, echoing the increasing medical needs of all Americans.[35]

This increase in the use of healthcare workers is not limited to seniors. A similar increase has been seen in the pediatric population. Lifesaving technologies have saved many children who would have died of their illnesses a few decades ago: micropreemies, children with multiple severe birth defects, and children with once-fatal genetic conditions, as well as older children who survived serious injuries and require ongoing care. A recent study found that between 1993 and 2005, the hospitalization rates for medically complex children (children with one or more medical conditions requiring specialty care) doubled.[36]

In addition, we are doing a better job of diagnosing and providing effective treatments for a variety of conditions. One such condition that we have gotten better at diagnosing is autism, diagnoses of which increased more than fivefold from 1996 to 2006. Each child with autism requires far more contact with healthcare professionals than most American children; they make multiple visits to pediatric neurologists, pediatric behavioral medicine specialists, and several types of therapists every year.

Another example of the increasing demand for health workers can be seen in this country's pediatric- and adult-obesity epidemics. *Epidemic* is not too strong a word. Since 1990, there has been a 76 percent increase in diabetes in adults 30 to 40 years old.[37] Thirty-four percent of all American adults and 17 percent of all American children are obese. People with obesity require multiple visits to physicians and nutritionists to lower their weight, in addition to seeing specialists for obesity-related health conditions, such as diabetes, cardiovascular disease, and joint damage.

The Downside of Health-Insurance Reform

On March 23, 2010, I felt as if I had awakened in a different country. My new country didn't deny medical coverage for people with "preexisting" conditions, didn't charge women more than men for health insurance based on gender alone, and didn't allow insurance companies to cancel your policy because you became severely ill.

In my opinion, health reform put us on the road to fixing our broken, costly healthcare system, but it is a double-edged sword. Healthcare reform will only increase the demands on the healthcare system and exacerbate our healthcare-worker shortage. Thirty-two million Americans who were previously unable to obtain or afford health insurance now will be able to. Ability to pay will no longer be *the* barrier to healthcare. Instead, the new barrier to healthcare will be the healthcare-worker shortage.

I am not the only one to come to this conclusion. After the passage of the Patient Protection and Affordable Care Act, both the American Medical Association (AMA) and the Association of American Medical Colleges (AAMC) analyzed the potential impacts and revised up their estimates of the current and future shortage of physicians in this country. Because more people will be able to buy health insurance and thus use the medical system, the AAMC has increased its prediction of the short-term physician shortage by 58 percent, from 39,600 to 62,900 in 2015.[38] Not only will health reform aggravate the shortage of primary-care physicians; the professional associations' analysis points out that it will worsen the specialist shortage as well.[39]

Beyond the sheer numbers of currently uninsured people whom the Affordable Care Act intends to help insure, many uninsured people are sicker than the general population and will require more services once they are insured. Many of the currently uninsured cannot qualify for or afford insurance precisely because they are chronically ill. Their lack of access to healthcare exacerbates this problem and worsens their conditions. When many previously healthy uninsured then become sick, they don't receive the care they need, and then they experience worse health status. According to one US health-system observer, this is a pool of patients with a lifetime of pent-up unmet medical need.

The state of Massachusetts offers a glimpse of what the United States may look like after health-insurance reform. In 2006, Massachusetts mandated that all residents obtain a minimal level of health insurance (subsidized for households that earned up to 300 percent of the federal poverty level) or pay a fine. Under the program, more than 340,000 people in that state were newly insured, and the demand on healthcare workers increased quickly and substantially. With hundreds of thousands of new patients entering the system with no offsetting increase in physicians, waiting times for new-patient appointments with an internist increased 58 percent—from 33 days to 52 days. *Half* of the primary-care practices in the state closed their doors to new patients, the highest level ever recorded in the state. For the first time, Massachusetts experienced a statewide shortage of primary-care workers. The shortages were worst in communities that already had shortages—communities such as Cape Cod and other vacation spots, where large numbers of seasonal workers were previously uninsured. But even Boston, with its many medical and nursing schools and hospitals, was affected.

A state with one of the greatest number of primary-care physicians per capita, Massachusetts experienced these shortages on expanding its health-insured population by just 5 percent. Adding 32 million people nationwide to health-insurance rolls over the next two to three years will increase the number of Americans with health insurance by a whopping 12 percent. We will surely see an even greater restricting of access to physicians after full implementation of the health-reform law.

Access to Healthcare

To complicate matters even further, the newly insured under health reform are more likely to live in medically underserved areas.

The healthcare-worker shortage is already far worse in rural America than in metropolitan America. While 20 percent of all Americans live in rural areas, only about 10 percent of the country's physicians and nurses work in these areas. The number of physicians per capita in metropolitan areas is 136 percent higher than that in rural counties; the number of dentists per capita is 150 percent higher.

In 2008—*before* Congress passed the health-reform bill—a survey of households in rural central Texas showed that nearly 25 percent of the insured older respondents had experienced difficulty getting an appointment to see a doctor in the past year. According to this survey, this one rural part of Texas will need an additional 3,000 doctors by 2020 to meet basic needs.[40] That was in 2008.

Another survey revealed that in rural Texarkana, at the border of Texas and Arkansas, patients wait 90 days to see a rheumatologist or neurologist. New primary-care patients have to wait three weeks to see a doctor. For Medicare patients, the wait can be even longer, since 58 percent of physician practices in this market have closed their doors to new Medicare patients.[41] A similar study in Indiana revealed that rural areas of the state were experiencing a shortage of almost every type of healthcare worker: physicians, nurses, physical therapists, mental-health counselors, pharmacists, social workers, health educators, speech pathologists, physician assistants, and psychologists.[42]

Delays in care are widely documented to worsen health outcomes. If you live far from providers' offices, as is the case in rural areas, a long delay can effectively mean *no access* to healthcare—whether you have health insurance or not. In its 2009 report titled *Health Status and Health Care Access of Farm and Rural Populations*, the USDA notes that rural populations experience higher mortality, disability, and chronic disease than their metropolitan counterparts, all aggravated by lack of proximity to healthcare.[43]

Since 2000, the number of times that hospitals have declared "no beds available" and temporarily stopped admitting patients has increased. "No bed available" doesn't mean a shortage of physical beds; it means not enough healthcare workers are available to take care of the patients in those beds. When I was working in the emergency room at the Children's National Medical Center, in Washington, DC—one of the largest pediatric ERs in the world and the regional coordinator for pediatric emergencies—the *closest open* pediatric bed at times was at King's Daughters Children's Hospital, in Norfolk, Virginia—200 miles and a three-and-a-half-hour drive away! At those times, critically ill children were either helicoptered or rushed by ambulance all the way to Norfolk.

Critically ill, chronically ill, or not, Americans are put at risk by increasing wait times at every stage of healthcare. A study conducted by Merritt Hawkins & Associates in 2009 revealed that wait times for nonurgent appointments in major metropolitan areas had increased in the past five years to an average of 50 days. Some of the highest wait times were for bread-and-butter specialists, such as family practitioners (63 days) and OB/GYNS (70 days).[44] These lengthening wait times to see a physician clearly indicate the effects of the health-workforce shortage on decreasing access to healthcare.

In 2005 the Commonwealth Fund conducted a survey of chronically ill patients in the United States, Australia, Canada, Germany, New Zealand, and the United Kingdom and found that *the United States ranked last* on several measures of access to and continuity of care. US patients were least likely to have a regular doctor; among those with a regular doctor, US patients were less likely to have had the same doctor for five years or more. US patients were more likely than patients in Canada, Germany, New Zealand, and the United Kingdom to report extreme difficulty in getting care at night or on weekends or holidays, unless they went to the local hospital's emergency department.

During the debate over healthcare reform, many people expressed understandable concerns over rationing of healthcare. The truth is, rationing is already here. What is being rationed is not drugs, tests, or medical procedures. Instead, what is being restricted is access to health workers who would offer these drugs, tests, or procedures. There are simply not enough health workers to meet the country's needs.

Supply and Demand, Accidents and Death

As we saw in the last section, the passage of healthcare reform has led health-policy experts to become concerned about the country's healthcare workforce and has led to longer waiting times to see physicians.[45] But what affect does this have on health? Generally, such research is hard to conduct in the United States, because the lack of universal health insurance makes it difficult to determine and quantify the non-insurance-related barriers to healthcare. Access to healthcare in the United States is greatly affected not only by whether or not people have health insurance, but by their specific insurance company, how many physicians accept that insurance, and what it covers. This makes it difficult to determine whether a given individual has poor access to healthcare due to lack of insurance or due to other factors, such as the shortage and maldistribution of healthcare workers.

But in countries that have universal health insurance, it is possible to directly study the effect of healthcare-worker shortages on health. A study released in 2010 in Canada, for example, showed that even when correcting for income, children living in Canadian counties with fewer primary-care physicians received less care and had worse health outcomes than children living in counties that had more primary-care physicians. The variation in access and outcomes was great. Some counties had as few as 1,720 children per primary-care physician (pediatrician or family practitioner); some had as many as 4,720 children per primary-care physician. As might be expected, the children living in the counties with fewer physicians had lower rates of primary-care visits (2.7 visits per child versus 7.5 visits per child). This included follow-up visits for new mothers, which are vital to monitoring the health of both baby and mother.[46]

Perhaps you saw *As Good as It Gets*, the 1997 movie in which Helen Hunt played a waitress with no health insurance and a young son with severe asthma. Without health insurance, she was unable to afford his asthma medicines; as a result, he had more frequent and more severe asthma attacks. And every time he had an asthma attack, she took him to the local emergency room. That movie scenario was based on fact: Children who do not have access to primary care, because of either lack of insurance or the shortage of healthcare providers, often use emergency rooms as a backup. In the Canadian study, the children in the counties with fewer primary-care physicians were 2.5 times more likely to visit the emergency rooms.

The Canadian study revealed significant health-service use and clinical-outcome differences for specific diseases, one of them asthma. In medical parlance, asthma is classified as an "ambulatory care sensitive condition," meaning that for people who suffer from this condition, the rate of hospitalization is directly dependent on the primary care they receive. Those who receive adequate primary care have lower rates of asthma complications and hospitalizations; those who receive inadequate primary care have significantly higher rates of both complications and hospitalizations.

For children, asthma is a major cause of missed school and hospitalization; it is highly reflective of the primary care the child is receiving. Children in Canadian counties with fewer physicians were 2.7 times more likely to go to the ER for asthma and were 1.6 times more likely to require hospitalization. Similar results were found for diabetes, another medical condition sensitive to adequate access to primary care.[47] Without adequate access to primary care, children with diabetes are much more likely to have their sugar levels spiral out of control, which can lead to a life-threatening condition called diabetic ketoacidosis—which can lead to coma and death if not treated immediately.

Delayed care from the health-worker shortage not only causes poor health and unnecessary suffering but also drives up healthcare costs. Prevention is generally cheaper than treatment. Primary care is generally cheaper than specialty care. Care given in physician offices is cheaper than care given in ERs or hospitals. People whose care is delayed are sicker when they eventually receive care, and the more severe the illness, the more costly the treatment.

The health-worker shortage also increases costs by driving up the wages of health workers faster than the rate of inflation. A large number of hospitals and clinics are chasing around a small number of workers, and they compete with each other by raising wages, a "rob Peter to pay Paul" situation that increases salaries without increasing the number of healthcare workers. The frequent staff turnovers that result mean that hospitals spend more money on recruiting and training new staff than they would if there were adequate numbers of healthcare workers.

In Los Angeles County, this kind of competition among county hospitals led to a 37 percent increase in the wages of nurse anesthetists in a single year.[48] According to Standard and Poor's, wages for healthcare workers in general have increased at a rate of 5 to 7 percent annually. These wage increases have occurred in an economic climate in which annual inflation has been less than 3 percent and in which national average wages have actually fallen.

Healthcare is one of the country's most recession-proof industries. Even in difficult times, many healthcare visits cannot be avoided, and even people who lack or lose their health insurance have a legal right to be seen in an emergency room. Health institutions rarely respond to decreased revenues by firing staff;

instead, they wring efficiencies out of their current staff and cut nonstaff "fat" out of their budget or reduce workers' hours. In many cases, rules on staffing ratios keep hospitals and nursing homes from laying off workers.

According to the US Bureau of Labor Statistics, the healthcare industry is the largest employer in the United States, employing roughly 14 million people. Ten of the 20 fastest-growing occupations are related to healthcare. By 2016, the healthcare industry will have generated 3 million new jobs in 10 years, more than in any other industry. These jobs represent 20 percent of all new US jobs over that period.

The healthcare industry has a job-growth rate of 22 percent, which is twice the predicted national job-growth average of 11 percent. The US Labor Department reported in March 2009 that, despite steep job cuts in nearly all other major industries, the healthcare sector continued to grow. In the previous month, during which a net of 681,000 jobs were lost, the healthcare sector added 27,000 jobs. That's more new healthcare jobs in a single month than the annual output of medical students in the United States.

Most health-workforce experts, myself included, believe that there has not been an intentional, coordinated effort to keep the stock of healthcare workers low. There are some prominent dissenters. Dr. Richard "Buz" Cooper, former dean of the Medical College of Wisconsin and current senior fellow at the Leonard Davis Institute of Health Economics, at the University of Pennsylvania, believes that Congress has purposely limited funding for medical and nurse education in an effort to keep the country's healthcare costs in check.[49]

Intentional or not, the negative impact on health is the same.

During the healthcare-reform process and anticipating the need for more healthcare workers, Congress proposed providing funding to increase the number of residency positions available in US hospitals by 15,000. The bill did not increase the number of medical school slots. Without additional med school graduates, how will these residencies be filled? Answer: by more than doubling our annual importation of foreign-trained doctors.

2

How the United States Created Its Healthcare-Workforce Problem

Our medical system has pioneered most major advances in health. Cancer vaccines, artificial hearts, whole-face transplants—American doctors and healthcare researchers are always on the cutting edge. So why can't we train the healthcare workers we need? There are several interrelated causes, but the fundamental reason is that the system is woefully fractured and disorganized. It is also extremely—and unnecessarily—expensive.

The university system in the United States is the envy of the world. In more than half a dozen global university-ranking systems, such as the Global Universities Rankings or the Academic Ranking of World Universities, the majority of the top ten universities are in this country. The United States has more educational institutions per capita than any country in the world. In terms of "tertiary enrollment"—the percentage of college-age people who are enrolled in college—we have the world's highest rate: 72 percent. And yet our state and locally run institutions are not training enough healthcare workers to meet our needs.

The United States did not decide as a matter of policy to create a healthcare system that relies on bringing in workers from the world's poorest and sickest countries rather than on training enough healthcare workers here. But over decades, through hundreds of decisions made by independent agencies operating in their own short-term interests, that is what has happened. Over time, we have developed a system so fragmented that it cannot perform the most basic function of training enough people to do this important work, let alone encouraging them to practice in the medical fields and geographic areas where they are most needed.

And because there is no communication among the various parts of the system—nor any central agency overseeing it to correct market failures—no one is working to solve this problem. For reasons as diverse as bureaucracy, cost, too much emphasis on research, and unnecessarily higher licensing standards (aka credential creep), a bad situation is growing more dire each year.

Bureaucracy Run Amok

The healthcare industry is the largest industry in the United States, comprising 16 percent of our economy. More than 580,000 establishments—hospitals, clinics, doctors' offices, pharmacies, health-sciences schools, medical-supply companies, pharmaceutical companies, insurance companies, nursing homes, research centers—make up the US healthcare industry. With huge variations in size, staffing patterns, and organizational structures,[1] they are responsible for assorted tasks within the system: training healthcare workers, providing health services, paying for health services, performing research, guaranteeing quality of care, protecting public health, and so on. And no one entity is overseeing or coordinating it.

These half-million-plus organizations are regulated by dozens of county, state, and federal government agencies, as well as independent agencies, that don't coordinate their actions and often don't even communicate with one another. Think of a country whose healthcare establishments are coordinated by a central agency, such as the British National Health Service. Then think of the polar opposite. That would be the United States. With no central coordination or oversight of the healthcare-system institutions, each regulatory organization is pursuing different goals, some of which are contradictory.

Just look at a partial list of the institutions that regulate my medical school, the Johns Hopkins University School of Medicine: the Liaison Committee on Medical Education, the Joint Commission on Accreditation of Healthcare Organizations, the Graduate Medical Education Board, the city of Baltimore, the state of Maryland, and several sections of the US Department of Health and Human Services. Trying to satisfy the disparate demands of these various regulators takes time, energy, attention, and money from the school's principal goal: training physicians.

As a physician practicing in the Washington, DC, area, I am regulated to exhaustion. I am licensed by the District of Columbia and the states of Maryland and Virginia through three separate boards and processes. My status as a pediatrician is regulated by the American Board of Pediatrics, whose board exam I must retake next year and whose byzantine quality-improvement program is so confusing that they have had to repeatedly delay its implementation. In addition, I am a fellow of my professional association, the American Academy of Pediatrics. I must regularly apply to the US Drug Enforcement Agency and the DC, Maryland, and Virginia Controlled Substance Registries for two types of certifications in order to prescribe controlled drugs; I maintain a personal identification number with the Centers for Medicare & Medicaid Services so that I can care for Medicaid patients; and I deal with dozens of individual insurance boards that must approve me to care for their patients. Every year, I have to take (and pay for) 30 hours of continuing medical education, despite the paucity of data to show that such formal continuing education improves health outcomes. Every year or two I have to turn in a record of a recent medical exam showing I am in good health and don't have tuberculosis. Every two years I have to be separately recertified in Neonatal Resuscitation and in Pediatric Advanced Life Support. Because I do locum tenens work, I have to maintain a panel of professional references who need to be contacted every time I do work for a new locum company.

It's practically a full-time job just keeping track of the paperwork. But the paperwork is not the main problem. With little or no communication among all these organizations, it's not surprising that actions that appear positive in one part of the system can have negative consequences in another part of the system. It is precisely this type of willy-nilly, uncoordinated regulation that has resulted in our health-worker shortage and led us to address the shortage in a manner that harms the United States and others.

Every year, about 42,000 people apply for the 17,000 first-year slots in US medical schools.[2] The country desperately needs more doctors, and there's clearly no shortage of bright young Americans interested in becoming physicians. But every year, some 25,000 young Americans have to consider other careers. That's because no one is minding the store. There's so little communication between medical schools, where physicians get their initial training, and hospital residency programs, where they get their final training, that we don't produce enough medical school graduates to fill the residency slots. Because there is little communication between the residencies and the eventual employers (hospitals, medical centers, and clinics), we don't produce enough physicians to fill job openings and meet community needs. Clearly, the market has failed.

If such a shortage occurred in an organized system, with good communication among all the institutional players, medical schools and residencies would be given the incentives or funds they need to train more doctors. The same story applies to the education of other healthcare professionals: Nursing schools, pharmacy schools, and so on are turning away tens of thousands of qualified applicants and not producing enough workers to fill job vacancies. Because our healthcare system is completely uncoordinated, employers have no say in either the number of graduates or the knowledge and skills they are taught.

The High Cost of Medical Training

Most physicians are trained by state medical colleges, which are run by the state governments or by independent boards over which the states have some control. Most nurses are trained by state colleges or community colleges, which are run by cities and counties. Local governments establish city and county hospitals and public-health services. States license healthcare workers. In short, the training of adequate numbers of healthcare workers is a state and local responsibility.

In a terrible conundrum, the states and communities that need healthcare workers most—especially southern and rural counties and states—tend to be the poorest. So the shortage of nurses and doctors is worst in the counties and states that have the fewest resources to train and retain them.

And now, of course, state and local governments must deal with ever-tightening budgets and increased costs. In 2001, amid spiraling costs, the Washington, DC, government shut down its only public hospital, DC General Hospital, after 200 years of service. That raised alarm among doctors, public-health leaders, and patients, who were concerned about access to healthcare for DC's large indigent population. But for every dramatic, attention-getting loss to a community's healthcare, there are hundreds of smaller, less publicized decisions—to cut or cap the number of healthcare workers trained, for instance—that cause little protest because few people notice. It's death by a thousand cuts.

One of the unintended side effects of the uncoordinated regulation of healthcare-training institutions is that it costs more to train healthcare workers in the United States than anywhere else, and it costs more to train healthcare workers than any other type of worker.

Educating an attorney or engineer in the United States costs about $100,000. It takes $200,000 to $300,000 to train a nurse. It's estimated that the real cost of training a physician in the United States is close to $1 million, about 50 percent more than it costs to train physicians in Europe. Students pay a portion of this through tuition and student loans, and the rest is paid for with federal and state funding directly to schools and subsidies provided by academic hospitals. The state of New York, for instance, each year provides more than $150 million in direct subsidies to its state medical schools.[3] Through Medicaid and Medicare, the US government provides subsidies directly to medical schools and to hospitals for physician education. Additional funding is given to state schools through the annual operational funding that states and counties give to universities and community colleges that train nurses and doctors. Many other groups provide grants and loans to institutions to subsidize healthcare-worker education: private foundations, philanthropists, and the training institutions themselves.

Students at private medical and nursing schools, such as those at Harvard and Johns Hopkins, pay exorbitant tuition—up to $50,000 per year—although tuition represents just a small fraction of the cost of their education. I received tens of thousands of dollars in grants and loans from Johns Hopkins, in addition to more than $200,000 in loans from the federal government and other lenders. The current average educational debt of medical students graduating from public and private medical schools is more than $150,000.[4] Even though salaries for doctors and nurses are among the highest in the country, it would be unreasonable to expect them to pay the full cost of their education. To do so would force almost all of them into higher-paying subspecialties and metropolitan practices, at the expense of desperately needed primary care, rural care, and lower-paid specialties, such as geriatrics. The United States already has a problem with overspecialization; we should never pursue a policy that makes it worse.

One reason it costs so much more to train doctors and nurses than non-health professionals is that for the most part, would-be lawyers and financial experts don't need much more than a professor in a classroom. Physicians and nurses in training demand much more extensive and expensive facilities and equipment: anatomy labs with cadavers and anatomical models; pathology labs with microscopes and slide sets (these alone start at tens of thousands of dollars); libraries filled with $200 books and $1,000 journals; paid "practice" patients on whom medical students train. (I still remember the poor woman on whom I performed my first pelvic exam. I'm glad she was paid!)

Physician education is particularly expensive due to the length of training, which exceeds that for all other professions: four years of undergraduate school; four years of medical school; and at least three years of residency, when a new doctor works under the supervision of senior physicians in, usually, a hospital or clinic. This minimum total of 11 years of higher education is longer than that required of physicians in most other countries. Most of the rest of the world requires five to six years of education before residency, not eight. And most countries require just one year, if any, of residency.

In addition, most people who enter medical school have to take years of prerequisites that have little to do with clinical work, which is what the vast majority of physicians do on a daily basis. These include calculus, physics, and chemistry.

Calculus? In today's world, you just need to be able to use a calculator. Physics? Perhaps understanding Brownian motion helped me appreciate how drugs diffuse through cells, but I could have learned about that in a 10-minute lecture rather than taking one year of physics that had more to do with the speed of boxes sliding on ramps and the interactions between neutrinos and positrons. Chemistry? Understanding acids and bases is helpful, but again, I could have learned that during a single lecture instead of taking one year of inorganic chemistry and one year of organic chemistry.

As an undergrad at Harvard, I was a biochemistry major (loved the intellectualism, hated the realities of a life spent alone in a lab) and took these prerequisite courses as an integral part of my major. But most of my pre-med classmates despised taking all those math and science classes and promptly forgot everything they had learned as soon as they turned in their final exams. So it is not surprising that performance in pre-med classes has been shown to be a poor predictor of success as a physician. Who would you rather have caring for you, a physician whose strong point was diagnosing and treating diseases of the human body, or one who was a star in physics and calculus?

These unnecessary or unnecessarily long prerequisites add years to a physician's training. It is estimated that these lost years of productivity, as well as the additional money spent on more years in school, and the increase in salaries needed to help repay medical school loans, cost the United States $25 billion per year.[5] There's no one watching the price of healthcare-worker education, because the institutions that regulate this education and drive up those costs are different from those that pay for the education. The institutions that regulate and pay for healthcare workers' educations are different from those that eventually pay the increased salary demands caused by the healthcare workers' needlessly large student debt.

Some medical schools have already started taking a rational look at their curriculum and reducing or eliminating classes that do not contribute directly to improving clinical practice. As we will discuss in more depth later in the book, there are now more than 10 medical school programs in the United States that offer a bachelor's degree and a medical degree in six or seven years rather than the standard eight years.

When Research Is a Bad Thing

I can tell you exactly when medical education became more expensive in this country than anywhere else in the world. It was in 1910, with publication of the Carnegie Foundation-funded Flexner Report.[6]

For decades, the American Medical Association had lobbied for the standardization of medical education in this country. At the turn of the last century, medical students were learning the trade in one of three basic ways: apprenticeship with a local practitioner, who offered hands-on instruction; a course of lectures at a medical college, from the physicians who owned the school; or a combination of didactic (lecture) and clinical training at a university and its affiliated hospital. Some wealthy students studied further at universities and hospitals in Europe. It would be an understatement to say that, due to both the heterogeneity of their educations and the near-lack of licensing exams, American physicians in the 19th and early 20th centuries varied greatly in their knowledge and abilities. No doubt patients suffered as a result.

So in 1904, the AMA created the Council on Medical Education, which, four years later, asked the Carnegie Foundation for the Advancement of Teaching to survey the country's medical schools. Abraham Flexner—a schoolteacher and educational theorist, not a physician—was selected for the task. After visiting all of the estimated 160 US medical schools, he decided that the best way to improve medical schools in the United States was to eliminate the majority of them. Flexner summed it up thus: "The point now to aim at is the development of the requisite number of properly supported institutions and the speedy demise of all others."[7]

The Flexner Report undoubtedly did some good in medical education: for example, requiring at least two years of college and then four years of medical school. It introduced the concept of evidence-based medicine and standardized curriculum. It called for higher admission and graduation requirements.

But the Flexner Report also had tremendous negative consequences. Universities had only just begun expanding female admissions, and that slim opening of that doorway immediately narrowed, greatly reducing the numbers of women—not to mention African Americans and other minorities—who were able to enter medical school. The Flexner Report forced the closure or consolidation of half the medical schools in the United States. Many of the schools forced to close were small schools in rural communities that trained young people from those communities and provided their residents with low-cost care. Perhaps the worst unintended consequence of the Flexner Report was that it turned most medical schools' attention away from the basic healthcare needs of their communities and focused it on research. The main goal of medical schools and the yardstick by which they were measured became research rather than patient care. This effect can be seen even today. A good example is my alma mater, the Johns Hopkins School of Medicine, which has pioneered many advances in health but is surrounded by a community with some of the worst health statistics in the United States. If you have ever watched the television show *The Wire*, you have seen the community in which Johns Hopkins is located. Johns Hopkins still does not have a family medicine department, because family medicine is seen as "not academic enough" for such a prestigious research institution. Yet family medicine doctors have been shown in study after study to be more likely to practice in underserved communities and provide care to the uninsured and underinsured. Medical research is important both to the advancement of health and to the American economy, but the vast majority of health workers work in patient care, so the emphasis of their training should be in patient care.

Moreover, as the *Journal of the American Medical Association* noted in 2004, "Although these reforms raised the quality of medical education in the United States, it concurrently caused a disproportionate reduction in the number of physicians serving disadvantaged communities: most small, rural medical colleges and all but two African American medical colleges were forced to close, leaving in their wake impoverished areas with far too few physicians. Furthermore, the increased entrance requirements and extended course of study now required to become a physician promoted 'professional elitism' and inhibited the economically underprivileged from pursuing careers in medicine."[8]

Just what I've been saying!

This overemphasis on research also unnecessarily drives up the cost of health-worker education. As we will discuss more in depth later, the more heavily involved a medical or nursing school is in research, the more expensive the internal and tuition costs of the education it provides. The need for research labs and nonteaching faculty drive up a school's infrastructure, salary, and overhead costs. These costs are not fully covered by research grants but instead are passed on the teaching hospital, the school, and the students.

The Johns Hopkins medical school prides itself on receiving more funding from the National Institutes of Health than any other institution in the country—but once I got to medical school, the worst and most irrelevant lectures I attended were given by scientists who, rather than teaching us something clinically relevant, just presented their current research.

To offer a particularly egregious example, my gross anatomy class was taught not by surgeons, who know how to navigate living anatomy, but by primatologists. Was this the best use of the school's money? We needed to learn relevant and medically useful information, such as which surface of the tibia to use, when necessary, for inserting an IV directly into the blood space within large bones. These well-intentioned anthropologists had us examine the bones of primates who walked on their fists and legs and compare them to the bones of primates who walked upright, to see which parts of the bones were enlarged to support the weight of the different muscles. We might as well have read about the work of Louis Leakey and Jane Goodall in Africa. It was fascinating, but hardly helpful. The university was using the medical students to subsidize its primatology research program.

The Real Causes of the Nursing Shortage

The emphasis on research made its way into the nursing profession, too. Before the 1950s, the majority of US nursing schools were located in hospitals. This system worked very well and is still widely used around the world. With hospital-based schools, nursing students got immediate, hands-on clinical experience, which has been shown to be more valuable than book learning in making good clinicians. Their contribution to the work of the hospital offset the cost of their education significantly, reducing the real cost of not only the nurses' education but also patient care. Since many of the nurses who graduated from a hospital nursing program ended up working for that hospital, the school and the future employer were the same, and the skills of the graduates matched the needs of the employer.

All that changed in 1948, when the Carnegie Foundation funded another study, the "Nursing for the Future" Report, also known as the Brown Report, which recommended that nursing schools be pulled out of hospitals and communities and placed in universities, to better integrate research into the curriculum.[9] This idea was good for academic nursing but terrible for clinical nursing, not to mention patients and their communities.

After the report came out, many hospital-based nursing programs shut down, and the rest moved to colleges, many of which did not have their own hospitals. This reduced access to hospitals and other clinical sites limited the number of nurses who could be trained and drove up the cost of training. With nursing schools no longer based within them, hospitals no longer had an incentive to let nursing students access their wards. Hospital-based nursing programs used the hospital's facilities and equipment, of course, while college-based programs had to build their own teaching space and buy their own equipment. In addition, hospital programs used the heavily experienced ward nurses to teach the students; these master nurses subsidized their teaching incomes with their clinical work, so the cost of instructors was minimal. College-based programs, however, had to come up with full-time salaries for their nursing professors.

The college-based programs began to require their nursing instructors to have master's degrees, which is unrealistic, given that registered nurses do not even have to have a bachelor's degree. This dramatically reduced the pool of eligible nursing professors. The requirement for a degree two levels above the standard qualification for a profession is unprecedented. You never hear about a shortage of medical school instructors or pharmacy instructors, because these professions require only the profession's baseline degree in order to teach.

When medical students or residents do clinical rotations in hospitals or clinics outside their medical school, they are supervised by the physicians who work in those clinics and hospitals. Many of these "community" physicians have unpaid adjunct-faculty positions or have received some training in how to supervise student doctors and do patient-based teaching. As a result, medical schools do not need to pay for additional faculty. But student nurses working at hospitals and clinics outside their nursing schools are not supervised by the nurses working in those facilities. Instead their professors from the nursing school travel to the facilities with them. This does more than radically increase staffing costs. The student nurses lose out on the wisdom of the experienced clinical nurses, and these master clinical nurses lose out on a potential career pathway in teaching. Medical schools, however, do integrate community physicians into medical school and residency, giving them adjunct positions and training in clinical mentoring so that they can be active participants in shaping the next generation of doctors. Considering that the profession excludes the majority of practicing nurses from being involved in nursing education, it is no wonder there is a shortage of nursing professors.

Indeed, one of the most significant reasons that nursing schools do not train more nurses is the lack of professors. Plenty of nurses are qualified to fill those positions, but the jobs just aren't attractive to them: Nurses with master's degrees, which most schools require of a nursing professor, can receive higher salaries performing clinical or management work. That's why so many nursing professorships sit empty.

The myth that young people don't want to become nurses due to low pay and poor working conditions is a powerful but incorrect argument for increasing nurses' wages. Since in the past, the majority of nurses have been women, many people assume the reason for the nursing shortage is that other career paths are now available to women.

It's true that as male-dominated careers have opened up to women, many smart, ambitious, high-achieving women who otherwise would have entered nursing have entered these newly available fields. However, the truth is that applications to US nursing schools have never been higher. We need at least 30,000 more nursing graduates per year—a 30 percent expansion. Some estimates bring the number to 90,000, a 90 percent expansion over current numbers.[10] Yet according to the American Association of Colleges of Nursing, in 2008 almost 50,000 qualified applicants to professional nursing programs, including nearly 6,000 people seeking to earn master's and doctoral degrees, were turned away because of the lack of openings.

When Higher Education Is a Bad Thing: Increased Requirements and Credential Creep

Another cause for the increase in the cost of healthcare-worker education is credential creep, which occurs as the various health professions seek to improve their professional images—and salaries—by raising their licensing requirements.

Audiologists offer the most egregious example of this nest feathering. Before 1990, most states required audiologists to have a minimum of a master's degree—that's six years of higher education in order to conduct hearing tests and place hearing aids. After intense lobbying, more and more states are increasing the requirement for a license to practice audiology to a doctorate. This means several more years of expensive tuition for the students, as well as an equivalent number of years of lost wages, money they did not earn because they were still in school.

Of course, to offer those doctoral programs, audiology schools need to hire more faculty, which increases both internal costs and tuition. With their higher academic degrees and the additional debt they incurred to gain them, audiologists have started demanding higher salaries. This cost is passed on to patients via higher health-insurance payments. The more worrisome cost is that requiring a doctorate to practice will reduce the number of audiologists, and thus reduce access to audiology services. Everyone wants to make more money, but it makes no sense to increase the costs for students and patients when it brings no cost-effectiveness in care.

Following the audiologists' lead, several other healthcare professions, among them occupational and physical therapists, have moved to make a doctorate their standard minimal degree for practice. As with audiologists, this will further increase the cost of their education and their care and further exacerbate the shortage of these healthcare workers. We even see this credential creep in the field of medicine, with the increasing interest in the "double-doctor," the MD/PhD. All of this drives up the cost of education and care while decreasing healthcare access and cost efficiency.

A similar movement has occurred among nurses, which is particularly concerning because nurses make up the largest part of the healthcare workforce. Until the 1990s, you could become a registered nurse through a two-year associate-degree program, a two- or three-year diploma program, or a four-year bachelor of science in nursing program. The associate and diploma programs focused more on hands-on delivery of care, while the bachelor's programs focused on theory. But over the past few decades, colleges have been shutting down their two-year associate-degree and three-year diploma programs. Why? Not because of the expense: Associate and diploma nursing programs are a faster and more cost-effective way to produce a registered nurse than bachelor's programs. Not due to a lack of applicants: In fact, associate and diploma programs are particularly popular with rural and minority students. Not due to licensing rates: Associate-degree and diploma nurses pass the certification exam at rates equal to those who attended bachelor's programs. The reason the schools are being closed is pressure from nurses with bachelor's degrees, who consider the value of their degree diminished by associate and diploma nurses.

Diploma programs used to be the dominant form of nursing education in the United States, with more than 800 such programs across the country. Now there are fewer than 100 programs, reducing the US production of nurses by tens of thousands each year and leaving many communities without a nursing school to provide them with a sustainable supply of nurses interested in practicing in their community. Associate and diploma programs are very popular with poor, rural, and minority communities: with poor communities because they are more affordable than university-based programs, and with rural communities because they are more likely to be located outside major metropolitan areas. Many people from these underserved communities are the first in their family to pursue postsecondary education, and without an experienced family member to guide them, they find the community-college programs easier to access. Eliminating these programs will further restrict these communities' access to nursing education and the number of nurses in the community. Given our expanding nursing and general healthcare-worker shortage, raising entry barriers to nursing is the *last* thing we should be doing.

Credential creep is also affecting nurse practitioners, a profession first created in Colorado to address the shortage of primary healthcare workers in rural and underserved communities. Primary care was the focus of their recruitment and training. For decades, this strategy was a success; nurse practitioners were more likely than physicians to practice in underserved communities, where they filled a needed role.

But as of 2015, the American Association of Colleges of Nursing will require newly graduating nurse practitioners to have a doctorate.[11] This will, of course, raise the barriers in terms of both time and financial investment. It will further restrict the number of people in rural and underserved communities who become nurse practitioners and will likely reduce the number that can be graduated each year. Data from medical school after medical school has shown that as the educational debt climbs, the student population tends to shift toward people from more affluent and metropolitan backgrounds, and that on graduation, these students are more likely to practice in metropolitan areas. As nurse practitioners position themselves as a doctorate-only profession, we are already seeing a shift in their practice sites: away from underserved areas and toward metropolitan areas, and away from primary care toward tertiary care in hospitals. In fact, in the last three years the number of nurse practitioners entering subspecialty fields has tripled.

Nurse practitioners were once seen as an answer to this country's primary-care shortage, but credential creep makes that highly unlikely. Unless the American Association of Colleges of Nursing reverses its decision and nurse practitioners return to their primary-care, underserved-community roots, a profession once considered a solution will become part of the problem.

The main justification for increasing the standard degree needed to practice a profession is that it improves the quality of care. It makes sense that the more years of training professionals have, the more knowledge and skills they will have on graduation. I accept this. Although associate degree and bachelor's degree nurses pass their licensing exams at the same rate, there is data that when all other things are the same, the patients of registered nurses with bachelor's degrees have better outcomes than patients of diploma nurses. But even with our growing health-worker shortage, this is not the question we are being asked as a country. We are not being asked, "Would you rather be cared for by an RN with four years of education or two years of education?" We are being asked, "Would you rather be cared by an RN with four years of education and 19 other patients or an RN with two years of education and only 9 other patients?" Or, if you live in an underserved community, "Would you rather be cared for by an RN with two years of education or no RN at all?" Our health workers are already of the highest quality in the world. The biggest health challenge we face as a nation is not the quality of our workers but the shortage of health workers. The Institute of Medicine report on medical errors does not cite the quality of health-worker preservice education as a significant issue. It does, however, cite systems problems, overwork, staff shortages, and high patient loads: "One of the report's main conclusions is that the majority of medical errors do not result from individual recklessness or the actions of a particular group—this is not a 'bad apple' problem. More commonly, errors are caused by faulty systems, processes, and conditions that lead people to make mistakes or fail to prevent them."[12] Associate-level RNs, master's-level physical therapists, and MD-level physicians are not "bad apples" that need to be phased out of our system.

I am also concerned that there has not been sufficient analysis of the cost benefit of credential creep. If we are going to increase the cost of education of almost all health professionals, what is the benefit in terms of improved health or money saved? If we double the cost of nursing education by eliminating two-year associates, what is the benefit? If we are going to invest even more money in our health system, is it really best spent in preservice training, the cost of which has been rising at twice the rate of inflation even without credential creep? Or would that money be better invested elsewhere in the health system, such as opening nurse clinics in rural areas, where they could screen patients for chronic diseases and help those already diagnosed better adhere to their treatment plan?

A Broken Admissions System

Many foreign-trained healthcare workers are brought to the United States specifically to address the maldistribution of healthcare providers. The main reason for the paucity of healthcare workers in rural and other underserved areas is that the admissions systems of our health-professional schools unintentionally select for people who prefer to live and work in metropolitan areas.

Admissions to medical school are heavily dependent on the Medical College Admission Test, or MCAT. The Association of American Medical Colleges (AAMC) developed this test with the well-intentioned notion that it would act as a standard benchmark against which to measure all applicants, regardless of their educational or social backgrounds. There was concern that grades are not truly reflective of achievement, or, rather, that the effort needed to get an A or a B can vary greatly. For example, earning a B in a math class at the University of Massachusetts may not represent the same level of achievement as a B earned in a math class at MIT.

The MCAT is a six-hour exam consisting of 221 multiple-choice and two essay questions. When researchers looked at how well this exam predicted students' success in the basic-science portion of medical school (the first two years), they found that the scores explained only 9 to 16 percent of the variance among students' grades. The MCAT scores proved even less helpful in explaining the variance of grades in the clinical portion of medical school (the second two years).[13]

A different set of researchers found that admissions interviews were more predictive of overall medical school performance.[14] Yet another team of researchers found that student psychosocial factors—such as personality, ability to communicate, and personal background—could explain 14 percent of the variations in students' clinical-competence scores, while their MCATs could explain only 4 percent.[15]

As a standardizing measure of knowledge, the MCAT is helpful. But significant evidence shows that the MCAT does not predict success in either medical school or as a physician. In the end, the MCAT scores are very sensitive to people's test-taking skills. Students who can afford to take private test-prep classes will do much better on the MCAT than poorer students who cannot afford such classes.

For the most part, what the MCAT measures is cognitive skills. Given the volume of ever-changing medical data that physicians need to understand and use on a daily basis, we do expect physicians to be the most intellectually strong members of the healthcare team. But good physicians need other skills and abilities, too. When patients are asked what characteristics they want in a physician, they say they consider thoroughness, communication skills, respectful behavior, emotional intelligence, and commitment to service as important as or more important than cognitive skills.[16] Sacrificing all the other qualities that make a good physician in order to select the most cognitively skilled for admission to medical school is not in the best interest of either medicine or the American people.

More Hoops, Higher Costs, Questionable Results

The various bodies that accredit health-professional schools and residencies have been imposing increasing requirements for accreditation. This, too, results in increased costs. Take, for example, the Liaison Committee on Medical Education (LCME), which accredits all the medical schools in the United States. With the exception of one patient advocate, the members of the committee are all from academic medicine.[17] There are no representatives from nonacademic providers of health services, which provide the majority of health services in this country. There are no representatives from groups that actually pay for the majority of health services, such as employers, insurance providers, and Centers for Medicare and Medicaid Services, the single largest payers of health services in the United States. Nor are there members of any private or public organizations that analyze the cost-effectiveness of medical care, such as the Agency for Healthcare Research and Quality or the National Association for Healthcare Quality.

As a result of this disconnect between the licensing committee, on the one hand, and the employers of physicians and producers and payers of healthcare, on the other, there is a huge discrepancy between the type of training the LCME mandates and the type of training that would allow us to produce adequate numbers of physicians. The LCME introduces requirements that create barriers to medical school, drive up the cost of physicians' education (and student debt), and have little documented cost-effective impact on patient care.

For example, a top-tier medical school was put on probation because of a new regulatory hoop. The LCME is requiring medical schools to track the details of specific types of patients the students have cared for and specific procedures the students have performed. There was no question about the quality of the school's graduates, who are some of the most esteemed and sought-after clinicians in the world; they advance the field of medicine through their work, pioneer lifesaving treatments, and win hundreds of National Institutes of Health grants each year. But the school encountered difficulty implementing the detailed tracking required, because every medical student's experience on clinical rotations is unique. Surely these new regulations were meant to improve the quality of graduates from medical schools on the bottom tiers, not to threaten the accreditation of top performers.

When I contacted the school administrators, I was told (on condition of anonymity) that the school had to hire four new staff members and an outside consulting company and buy expensive software just to track the required information. They had to hire dozens of professional actors to act as "standardized patients." The cost and complexity of the system put in place to satisfy the regulations will make it more difficult to expand the medical school program and drive up the cost of attending the school—with little evidence of improving health outcomes.

The people I spoke with expressed concern that new LCME rules were making the curriculum more rigid; now the school could not choose to put greater emphasis on primary care. According to one of the administrators, a graduate of the medical school for which she worked, "the quality of the education has been marginally improved, but the flexibility, creativity, and imagination of the education have been greatly reduced as a result of the new regulations. These regulations are driven by small scandals rather than evidence." In sum, rather than having their intended effect of improving the quality of medical school graduates, the new regulations seem to be driving up the cost and decreasing the quality of the graduates.

Improving quality of care is an admirable goal. However, most evidence suggests that quality of care is best improved at the point of care, not at the education level. *Most medical errors don't occur because a healthcare worker did not know something.* They occur because clinics and hospitals do not have the proper support and safety systems in place—which includes having enough healthcare workers on staff. Experts largely agree that health outcomes in the United States are far below those in European countries not because of the quality of care provided to patients that receive care, but because of the limited access (in numbers or location) to healthcare providers and the large numbers of people who therefore receive minimal or no care.

Public versus Private

So far I have focused on how the United States unnecessarily constrains the number of Americans who can be trained as healthcare workers, bringing in tens of thousands of foreign healthcare workers each year instead. But it gets worse. Demand among young Americans for training in the healthcare professions is so strong that many actually go *overseas* to receive an education, and then return to the United States to practice. So now we're even outsourcing the education of our young people. Will *anything* be made in the United States anymore?

Rather than expanding enrollment or opening more health-professional schools, we are sending some US citizens to non-

US-accredited medical schools in other countries. In 2008 the US Department of Education spent $315 million in student loans for American citizens studying healthcare in other countries. Although at least this money went toward training Americans, it would have been better spent on opening more schools—especially nursing schools—in this country. But rather than staying in the United States, where it would have created jobs, the money was absorbed into the economies of other countries.

The reality is, we have made the cost of a health-professional education so expensive that neither the students nor the states nor the federal government can or wants to foot the bill to train enough workers to meet our needs. In general, the cost of higher education has been increasing at a rate of 8 percent a year—faster than inflation and wages—but the cost of educating healthcare workers has been increasing even faster.[18]

Every year, 25,000 residency slots open in American hospitals, but only 16,000 medical school graduates are available to fill them. In other words, every year, US medical schools could graduate 9,000 more doctors guaranteed to find jobs. I am a believer in the power of private markets. So why don't we train them in the private sector? The answer is that with the current misaligned regulatory environment, even private schools can't make medical and nursing education pay.

The number of private not-for-profit and private for-profit universities has mushroomed in the last few years. These schools keep costs low by focusing on academics rather than on sports and extracurricular activities and often rent rather than own facilities. Growth has been particularly strong among for-profit schools; names such as Walden, DeVry, and Strayer University are becoming well known. Apollo Group, Inc., which owns the University of Phoenix, is even publicly traded. But not one of these for-profit universities has a medical school—because it's too expensive.

Although healthcare in the United States is provided chiefly through the private sector, the doctors and nurses who deliver this care are produced through public subsidies. Unlike in a country like Britain, with its National Health Service, the United States has no system linking the provision of healthcare to the production of the caregivers. Training, payment for training, need for workers, and hiring is utterly uncoordinated; there is no way to indicate any shortage or surplus of workers. Hospitals in need of doctors and nurses have no mechanism for asking the education system to produce them.

In short, we have a public-sector-driven education system producing healthcare workers at a higher and higher cost, and a private-sector market-driven job arena that is pushing for lower and lower wages. In the meantime, while the percentage of Americans with higher education has increased, the number of doctors and nurses trained in the United States each year has stagnated since the early 1980s, and the ratio of graduates to the total population has fallen. We are making up the shortfall with less expensive, foreign-trained healthcare workers.

The Path to America

Every year, tens of thousands of foreign-trained doctors, nurses, and other healthcare providers arrive in the United States. Even if they work in rural and poorer communities, the places they are needed most, they don't tend to stay there. And in many cases, the unregulated, multibillion-dollar recruiting industry abuses them and endangers their lives. Yet few people are aware of how they are recruited, how they get here, and what they do once they arrive.

It was March 18, 1999, my residency Match Day. With my 120 classmates, I sat in the Johns Hopkins medical school auditorium, holding a sealed white envelope. At precisely noon, we opened our envelopes and found out where we would start our first paid work as physicians and spend the next three to six years of our lives. The envelopes contained the names of the medical residencies with which we had been "matched." My envelope contained good news. I was to go to Children's National Medical Center, a top-ranking children's hospital in Washington, DC, the epicenter of my chosen field, global health.

Unbeknownst to me or my medical school classmates, thousands of physicians outside the United States were also getting their match news that day. Medical schools in the United States do not produce enough physicians each year to fill all 25,000 residency slots. Each year, just 16,000 or so medical students graduate from US medical schools; so each year, around 9,000 foreign-trained doctors are given earmarked visas and brought into the country to fill the rest of the residencies. These positions are so sought after that more foreign medical school graduates apply to the US residency match than there are students graduating from American medical schools. Domestically trained medical students are in such short supply that the foreign medical graduates have a 40 percent chance of matching to a residency position—with a guaranteed visa, of course.[1]

A full one-quarter of the physicians in this country have been imported from elsewhere—an increase of 160 percent since 1975. Immigrant physicians account for 27 percent of the country's 96,937 residents and medical fellows. (Medical fellowships are high-level training programs that enable physicians to specialize even further after residency.)[2] As for nurses, 10,000 foreign nurses are newly licensed in the United States each year—taking the place of 10,000 Americans who will never be able to enter the nursing profession.[3] Exact data are not available on the percentage on foreign-trained workers in the other healthcare professions, but given the number of visas given to foreign-trained healthcare workers each year, these professions likely have a similar proportion of foreign-trained workers. And every year, foreign-trained healthcare workers make up a greater percentage of the healthcare workers in the United States.[4]

It is no accident that more than one-quarter of our healthcare workers are imported labor. Behind this phenomenon is a multibillion-dollar international healthcare-worker recruitment business. This industry is so large that the US-based international recruiters report operations in 74 countries, with plans for further expansion. More than half of the international health-worker recruitment agencies polled in 2007 indicated that they planned to expand their activities to even more countries. Despite its size, this industry keeps a very low profile, and most

Americans—even most people working in the healthcare sector—are completely unaware of its existence.

The International Doctor-Recruitment Industry

The medical-resident job market in the United States is unlike any other job market in the world. Every year on June 30, at the stroke of midnight, around 25,000 senior residents in US hospitals and clinics complete their residencies and graduate. On July 1, 25,000 new residents must replace them to keep our hospitals and clinics running. In other industries, from banking to manufacturing, loss of workers happens gradually, and workers can be replaced over time. But in the medical-resident industry, virtually all attrition and hiring happens on a single day.

It's not feasible for US residencies to make offers to their preferred candidates, wait to hear how many of those offers are accepted, and extend additional rounds of offers until all the medical-resident slots are filled. But failure to fill even a few of the residency spots would leave hospitals unable to care for their usual number of patients at an acceptable level of quality. In order to make this mass-hiring process manageable, an independent corporation, the National Resident Matching Program, was established in 1952 to run "the match."

All foreign doctors who enter the United States, no matter how senior, must do a minimum of one year of residency to receive a US medical license and become a general practitioner. Very few medical-malpractice companies will insure the services of general practitioners. So most physicians want to become board certified in a specialty, such as pediatrics, internal medicine, or surgery, which means they complete full residencies of three years or more.

Just as I did, just as all American medical students do, foreign doctors apply for residencies through the National Resident Matching Program. After interviewing with the hospitals most interested in them, the graduating students pay a fee to the NRMP and rank the residency programs in order of preference. The hospitals, too, pay a fee and list the applicants in order of preference. It is like a complex dating game. The NRMP uses a computer algorithm to develop the best systemwide matches of residencies and applicants. In March of every year, these matches are mailed out, and the applicants discover where they will be doing their residencies.

Every year, the NRMP fills the 25,000 residency positions from a pool of 36,000 applicants. Of these applicants, a majority—about 20,000—are foreign-trained physicians.

With 36,000 applicants for 25,000 positions, this means that each year more than 10,000 match applicants do not receive a match, generally because they had lower grades from less prestigious programs and/or did not apply to enough residencies or enough less desirable "fallback" residencies. These men and women participate in the "scramble," the shotgun wedding of the medical world. This is how unmatched applicants and residencies with empty slots are brought together. Most of the residency programs that are left with empty positions and have to participate in the scramble are the primary-care programs in rural areas, and the majority of the applicants who scramble are foreign-trained doctors.

As you can imagine, competition for the 9,000 slots that can't be filled by US med school graduates each year is fierce. Many foreign applicants try to improve their attractiveness for the match by engaging the services of companies that promise to improve their chances. A few companies do seem to provide a reasonable service to those physicians, but some companies prey on their hopes and engage in ethically questionable behavior. For fees as high as $5,000, these companies make a variety of largely unsubstantiated claims. For instance, one company, FMG America, advertises, "We ensure U.S. medical placement for all qualified candidates."

Many of these companies claim that a foreign-trained physician can improve his or her match chances through a volunteer "observership" in a US hospital or clinic. As its name implies, this practice involves watching a US-licensed physician conducting his or her hospital or clinical practice, following him or her through the day and sitting in on patient interactions. But the foreign doctors who sign on for observerships are neither licensed to practice medicine nor enrolled in a US medical school or residency. They cannot care for patients, develop treatment plans, or write prescriptions or medical orders, so it is hard to say what practical benefit the observerships provide.

The companies that recruit foreign doctors for US residencies do not sit back and wait for the doctors to come to them. They place ads in the medical journals in developing countries; some companies even place ads on Craigslist, claiming to be able to help foreign doctors get into US residencies.[5]

Some physician-recruitment companies will write letters of recommendation for a fee—hardly an ethical practice. Others claim they can "polish" the résumés and personal statements of foreign doctors, which certainly raises doubts about the veracity of the résumés and whether the personal statements reflect the true thoughts and writing abilities of the applicant. Some companies promise to submit applications through "alternative channels"—that is, other than through the National Resident Matching Program—although no such channels legally exist. Even if these companies do have personal relationships with residency directors and can direct attention to their clients' applications, this is not an ethical practice. They claim to be able to find out which residency programs might be interested in the applicant before he or she submits a formal application to the NRMP; again, even if they can do this, it is not ethical.

The recruitment companies help foreign doctors practice for the match interviews and get the tourist visas needed to come here for those interviews. They even help write thank-you notes. If a foreign-trained physician needs that much help getting a residency position, he or she is probably not the person you want caring for you. Residency slots and the privilege of practicing medicine in the United States should be earned, not purchased.

Because foreign-trained medical doctors are not familiar with the US system, they are quite vulnerable to unethical practices and fraud. Foreign doctors who have complained about these companies have said, for example, that no services were provided or that the services were of such poor quality that they were useless. According to one online complaint, "FMG America doesn't provide you with any real externships, just telephone numbers of individuals. Dr. Cohen, one of the guys who is supposedly working for you, tells you to never give information about FMG America to the individual with whom you are trying to get an externship. . . . They use fear tactics to prevent IMGs [International Medical Graduates] to never contact agencies to help them get their money back."[6] Complaints have been filed with the US Better Business Bureau, which gives FMG America an F rating. Several of these physician-recruitment companies, among them IMGresidency.com and FMGamerica.com, have been investigated for fraud or sued by foreign doctors who claim to have been scammed.[7] Unfortunately, these companies are still operating.

To offset the problem of physician-recruitment companies preying on foreign-trained physicians, the Educational Commission for Foreign Medical Graduates—the independent body that certifies foreign-trained physicians for entry into this country—offers official advisory services to all foreign medical school graduates through its International Medical Graduates Advisors Network.[8]

Life does not get much easier once a foreign-trained doctor has made his or her way into a US residency. Chat rooms and blogs for foreign-trained doctors, such as IMG Digest (tagline: "coz every medical student is a potential IMG")[9] are full of stories of abuse of foreign-trained doctors in residency programs: lower wages than US-trained residents, weekly hours over the legal 80-hour limit, patient loads beyond recognized standards, abusive and manipulative program directors.

In the less attractive rural residencies, it is not unusual to see attrition rates among foreign physicians of 50 percent. Foreign residents are more likely to be terminated due to poor performance than US-trained residents. They are also more likely to report that they are leaving a residency due to unfairly low wages, overwork, or abusive residency directors. In 2009, imgforum.com, a website on which foreign-trained resident physicians can report abuse, had 29,000 individual posts with stories about discrimination, and another 14,000 posts about firings for poor performance.

Data on physician disciplinary action is more readily available from Britain's centralized National Health Service than in the United States, which has more than 50 different state and territory medical boards, each of which keeps independent records. In the British system, while foreign-trained doctors are just as likely as their domestic-trained counterparts to face initial disciplinary review, foreign-trained doctors are twice as likely to face subsequent disciplinary hearings. They make up two-thirds of the physicians whose licenses are revoked.[10] The license revocations are for both technical and ethical violations, from clinical incompetence and patient endangerment to sexual misconduct and selling prescription drugs.

There also have been cases of foreign-trained physicians showing significant ethical lapses, raising concern that medical ethics may not be appropriately emphasized in non-US medical schools. One high-profile case in this country centered on Dr. Yasser Awaad, an Egyptian-trained neurologist who practiced in the Dearborn, Michigan, area. He was accused of falsely diagnosing dozens of children with epilepsy and charging their insurance companies for very expensive treatments, from which he profited greatly.[11] He went so far as to implant brain-stimulating devices into patients who did not need them. Cases such as this one raise serious questions about the type of screening and orientation foreign-trained physicians receive before they start practicing in the United States.

The International Nurse-Recruitment Industry

The nurse-recruitment industry is far larger and more complex than that for medical residents and doctors. Not only are more nurses imported every year; in addition, there is no equivalent of the match for nurses. And whereas all doctors must enter through an academic hospital, nurses can enter the United States through employment at a multitude of different institutions, including community-based clinics, nursing homes, public health agencies, and every type of hospital. The international nurse-recruitment industry began innocently enough soon after World War II, as war brides of American soldiers saw an opportunity to bring to the United States family members and friends who were nurses in their home countries. Many of these women saw a chance to make some money at the same time. The process began through informal networks, but with no regulations, nurse-recruitment businesses quickly sprang up and became immensely profitable.

By the 1960s the nurse-recruitment industry had expanded beyond passive recruitment of friends and family. The process gradually became more aggressive, to the point where in many African countries, recruiters set up tables at nursing school graduation ceremonies. It is not too much to say that global recruiting changed the school and work environment from one in which a nurse made an active decision to emigrate to one in which she has to make a conscious decision *not* to leave. Ann Phoya, the planning director for the Malawian Ministry of Health and the former chief nursing officer, jokes that she should have moved her office to the national airport, because that is where the nurses were. Today, nurses in developing countries are so bombarded with proposals to migrate that they must, on a regular basis, decide to stay home.

The Commission on Graduates of Foreign Nursing Schools reports that the number of countries from which nurses applied to take the National Council Licensure Examination (NCLEX)—the computer-based exam that all foreign-trained registered nurses and foreign-trained licensed practical nurses must pass to be licensed in the United States—expanded from 90 in 1983 to 139 in 2005.[12] The significance of this trend is that recruiters moved from large middle-income countries like the Philippines and Mexico, which have relatively large pools of nurses, to smaller and poorer countries from which the loss of a few hundred—even a few dozen—nurses can cause a huge difference in the availability and quality of healthcare.

Because of the well-documented "escalator" effect, even recruiting nurses from middle-income or wealthy nations can cause tremendous problems in all countries. A nurse who cannot emigrate to the United States because her NCLEX scores are too low may get a job in Poland and improve her skills there, then move to the United Kingdom, retake the NCLEX, and eventually come to the United States. Or she may stay in the United Kingdom to replace a UK nurse who immigrated to the United States. Since many other wealthy countries have nursing shortages, taking nurses from them hurts their healthcare systems as well or forces them to recruit from poorer countries.

Norway's foreign nurses, for instance, tend to come from Eastern Europe, where native-born nurses are generally replaced with those from developing countries. Norway has provided global leadership on the healthcare-worker shortage, both through diplomacy and by funding research on the issue. Having recently experienced a scandal over the care of seniors by foreign nurses, the Norwegian government is redoubling its efforts and has required all government ministries, including ministries of health, labor, and defense, to work together on the problem. It is considering banning all foreign recruitment of nurses.

In the United States, the nurse-recruiting industry has grown almost tenfold, from 30 to 40 companies in the 1990s to more than 267 in 2007. This rapid growth reflects the deepening nursing shortage—the need to import more foreign nurses just to provide basic health coverage. The demand for foreign nurses has also increased because of another aspect of the nursing shortage: increased turnover. As more and more hospitals compete for the same number of domestically trained nurses, they often try to lure nurses with higher salaries, better hours, or expanded benefits. Domestically trained nurses do not work long at the same facility anymore; they move on when they receive a better offer from another hospital.

This rapid turnover increases the need for substitute nurses as the hospitals search for a full-time replacement. Foreign-trained nurses are often brought into the country to perform this temporary role. As the nursing shortage worsens, not only does the number of nurses needed grow, but the amount that hospitals are willing to pay a recruiting company for a nurse also rises. This increases both the per capita profits and the total potential profits a recruiting company can make, based on the volume of nurses they import. As more recruiting companies enter the field and competition increases, the companies may resort to even more aggressive tactics, recruit less-qualified nurses, and recruit more nurses from countries with severe shortages of healthcare workers.

Recruiting Nurses Equals Big Business

As the money to be made importing foreign-trained nurses grew, so did the number of recruiting companies. Defining the industry's scope is challenging, though, because the lack of standards means that recruiters are doing business under a variety of labels: broker, facilitator, handler, intermediary. In addition, many large hospitals, academic centers, and nursing homes run their own recruiting agencies. They do so under their own business licenses rather than recruiter-specific licenses, so the number of nursing recruits coming to this country under their auspices is extremely hard to track.

International nurse-recruiting agencies use three recruitment models. The most basic is the *placement* model. This type of agency signs a contract with a hospital to manage the recruiting, credentialing, licensing, and immigration process for a specified number of foreign nurses. The nurses have a temporary contract with the recruitment agency, but shortly after their arrival in the United States, they sign a contract with the hospital and join its staff.

Both hospitals and nurses prefer working with placement

agencies. Hospitals like it because it is cheaper for them: They pay a lump-sum fee up front and gain a nurse who will be with them for more than a few days or weeks. Nurses prefer it because staff nurses tend to be treated better than agency nurses—they receive training from the hospital and are given preferred assignments. Smaller recruiting agencies favor the placement model because it is the easiest to implement and requires the least investment and organizational capacity.

As agencies get larger, they tend to move to a more lucrative form of organization. About 45 percent of the international nurse-recruiting companies use the *staffing*, or agency, model. Here, the nurse remains the employee of the agency even after she arrives in the United States. The agency places the nurse as a temporary substitute in, for example, a hospital, which pays the agency to replace sick or vacationing nurses or plug vacancy holes while the hospital looks for a permanent nurse. No matter how pleased the hospital might be with the foreign nurse, it can't hire her because of her long-term contract with the recruiting company.

As long as she remains employed with the agency, the nurse is a revenue stream. Rather than making a few thousand dollars in a one-time transaction, as the placement agencies do, the staffing agencies can make tens or hundreds of thousands of dollars off a single recruit. Instead of charging an up-front fee, the agency takes a cut of the larger fee they charge the hospital. The hospital pays the agency at a rate twice the hourly salary of a staff nurse; the nurse gets a standard salary; and the agency makes a profit of about $50,000 per year—for each nurse.

Despite the higher price of "agency" nurses, some hospitals use them because they cannot pay the lump sum required for recruiting a staff nurse. For the hospital the staffing-model expense is spread over months or years, while the nurse is working, rather than being borne before the nurse enters the country. Needless to say, increasing the hospital's costs increases our healthcare costs.

Many recruiters consider the staffing model unethical, because it keeps nurses rotating through unfamiliar environments.[13] Moving so frequently from one substitute position to another, the foreign nurses are unable to build up the professional networks and long-term experience and references they need to get a job outside the recruiting company. Their contracts tend to last several years and have buyout provisions that make it difficult for them to leave the agency. These contracts and the lack of professional networks and references effectively trap them in their agency jobs. The frequent rotation of the foreign nurses also poses a safety risk, because they are constantly practicing in a new environment, with different procedures and rules and different types of patients.

The third model of recruiting is known as the *direct* model, because it is used by major hospital systems and academic centers that have decided to cut out the middle man and recruit foreign nurses themselves. By doing their own recruiting, they can reduce their costs, and their name recognition and guaranteed location ensure that they can recruit the best nurses.

Because these centers often hire hundreds of nurses a year thanks to staff turnover, they have the volume and the in-house human-resources staff to reach economies of scale that make it worthwhile to do their own recruiting. One study done in the Philippines showed that the academic centers have a major advantage over the stand-alone recruiting agencies. Nurses who sign with a placement or staffing agency know they have no guarantee regarding placement and will most likely end up in a rural area or a nursing home. Nurses who sign with a major hospital or an academic center with a good reputation know the city and facility in which they will be working, as well as the quality of the institution.

The hospital and academic centers' percentage of market share has increased greatly. Stand-alone recruitment agencies report signing up just a few more foreign nurses than were recruited directly by hospitals and academic centers.[14] As they become more proficient in recruiting—and begin to view international nurse recruiting as a source of income—many hospital-based recruiting agencies offer their services to smaller hospitals that cannot afford to do their own recruiting.

A smaller number of nurses enter the United States using the services of immigration-law firms. Many such firms specialize in healthcare-worker immigration, performing the services the recruitment and placement agencies do. This includes providing assistance in applying for the visa, locating and applying for a specific job, and gaining professional certification. A nurse might choose to use a law firm rather than a recruiter if she has enough money to pay the firm up front and wants more control of the situation—if she has a specific city in mind, for instance. Immigration-law firms range from single-lawyer practices working locally to organizations such as Southern California–based Global Law Center (whose website says its office staff speaks Spanish, Farsi, Hindi, Tagalog, Urdu, and Punjabi) to multicountry law firms such as Siskind Susser, which, in addition to law offices in the United States and Canada, maintains affiliate offices in Tijuana, Buenos Aires, and Beijing.

Even some domestic and international recruiters that previously had not been recruiting nurses overseas have now entered the business. A new class of entrant is the IT (information technology) recruiting company, such as DB Healthcare, with an office in Boston and several offices in India. As the tech sector continues to deflate and the healthcare sector expands, the latter looks more and more like a good replacement business. With offices and professionals all over the world, IT-recruiting agencies can easily make the switch. Often, the IT companies take a shortcut and simply buy a nurse-recruitment agency.

Many big recruiting agencies have responded to the competition by consolidating and growing larger still. Smaller recruiting firms are being bought by larger ones. As the preferred business model shifts from placement to staffing, small recruiting companies need access to larger amounts of capital, so they are often unopposed to being purchased.[15] Cross Country Staffing, with annual revenues of $115 million, and AMN Healthcare, with annual revenues of $173 million, are two of the five international nurse-recruitment firms that are so large they are publicly traded.[16]

Some agencies bring in 800 or more nurses a year. Most often, a healthworker-recruiting firm will buy another to gain entry into a growth country, such as India or the Philippines, two of the world's largest suppliers of nurses. Clearly, this consolidation will lead to a shift from the placement model to the staffing model, with even more foreign nurses being used as substitutes.

Recruitment-Agency Services

What are recruitment agencies doing for the $15,000 to $25,000 the client hospitals pay for each foreign nurse? First, they locate the nurses. They advertise in newspapers and online, but far more often they contact nurses at career fairs, via union and nursing-council meetings and publications, and at the healthcare facilities in which they work. Most controversially, they set up relationships with nursing schools and contact nurses as they graduate, even while they are still students.

Foreign-nurse recruiters talk about potential salaries in the United States that are 10 to 20 times higher than salaries in the nurse's country. They discuss educational opportunities for the nurse and her family. They tout the ease with which someone on a nurse's salary can buy a home. Some of their more aggressive behavior has spurred an international debate over "active recruitment." When are recruiters helping nurses realize a dream of working in a wealthy country, and when are they planting, even selling, that dream?

Once it has recruited a nurse, the agency must determine that she has the education and work experience she claims to have. This is known as credentialing. Once it has verified her nursing degree and grades and has talked with her employer to ascertain her years of employment, experience, and performance, the agency helps her obtain her US nursing license. This involves helping her enroll in and study for the NCLEX, the exam that all foreign-trained registered nurses and foreign-trained licensed practical nurses must pass.

The agency helps the nurse put together a formal résumé and fill out state-license application forms. Then it finds a hospital interested in hiring the nurse. It completes all the forms, collects supporting material for the visa, and guides the nurse through the entire Byzantine process. The agency helps the nurse make her travel arrangements. Some agencies purchase her airline ticket and others even provide housing and orientation once the nurse arrives in the United States.

Payment for and comprehensiveness of the service can vary widely. Many agencies ask the nurse for a "placement fee" up front; others collect the fee once she is working in the United States. Some agencies collect the fee from the hiring hospital.

The time between the request for a nurse from a hospital, nursing home, or clinic and the nurse's first day on the job also varies. US-trained nurses are usually already licensed in the state in which the hiring hospital is located; if not, they can quickly obtain a nursing license for that state. But foreign-trained nurses, even with recruiting agencies to help them, can spend months navigating the complexities of the US visa system; the whole process can take anywhere from 18 months to more than four years. Needless to say, this long turnaround time does not meet the greatest need in the fastest-growing sector of the US healthcare industry—the need for more nurses.

Unethical Recruiting Practices

Nurse-recruiting firms do not have to follow any standards or code of ethics. US-based firms merely have to have a business license in the state in which they are based; there's no oversight of their activity at the state or federal level. This lack of standards, in a setting of extreme power and knowledge imbalance between the foreign nurses and the international recruiters, has led to many illegal and unethical practices. The International Council of Nurses, the global professional association for nurses, has denounced many recruitment practices, saying they "exploit nurses or mislead them into accepting job responsibilities and working conditions that are incompatible with their qualifications, skills, and experience."[17]

Indeed, some recruiting agencies are downright scams. One American hospital reports paying more than $100,000 in recruiting fees and having received not a single nurse.[18]

And sometimes a nurse is conned into spending her life's savings and getting nothing in return. Many experts who study the recruitment industry consider taking any money from the nurses unethical, because the hospitals are already paying recruiting fees, and the nurses are not guaranteed a job. Collecting fees from nurses—the practice of 18 percent of foreign-nurse recruiters—has been banned in the United Kingdom. In the United

States, it is illegal to collect such up-front fees when recruiting migrant farmworkers, yet it is still legal when recruiting nurses.

US labor law does state that foreign nurses should receive the prevailing wage for their work. But surveys of foreign nurses who work as hospital temps for staffing agencies indicate that they regularly receive less than US nurses who work on a hospital staff. Reported substandard wages are as low as $10 per hour less than the prevailing wage. Foreign nurses also report being paid only their regular hourly wage for overtime—a direct violation of US labor law. They are often paid late or for fewer hours than they worked.

Some staffing agencies reportedly set wages by nationality—paying nurses from South Korea, for instance, more than nurses from the Philippines, a poorer country. Most companies that recruit both in the United States and internationally keep the two business lines separate, which makes it easier to offer different wages and working conditions to domestic and foreign nurses. Other unethical practices include altering contracts without the nurse's permission and withholding green cards. Green cards are supposed to be given to a person as soon as they have been issued. They are not meant to be held as collateral to assure that a nurse honors her contract.

Once an agency with a staff business model recoups its investment costs in bringing the nurse to the United States, any additional time she works greatly increases its profit, because the agency earns a commission for every hour its nurses work. So agencies have pressured nurses to work more than the usual overtime; if the nurse refuses, she may be threatened with a phone call to immigration authorities.

Some agencies require foreign nurses to commit to contracts of up to three years. If the nurse breaks the contract for any reason—a family emergency back home, inability to function in the high-pressure environment of American hospitals, culture shock—she must pay a "breach" fee of from $10,000 to $50,000. It must be paid in a lump sum—no installments are accepted. A US-trained healthcare worker, in her own country and working in an environment with which she is familiar, might find this practice acceptable and might be able to afford the breach fee. But how can a nurse who at home makes $1,000 a year ever pay such a high fee? She is a virtual prisoner of the recruiting agency.

The most famous example of abuse of foreign nurses is the "Sentosa 27" case. The Sentosa Recruitment Agency brought 27 nurses and a physical therapist to New York from the Philippines, promising them permanent hospital jobs. Instead, the nurses were placed in substitute positions in various nursing homes. (Sixty-one percent of foreign-licensed practical nurses end up in nursing homes, where they do low-level tasks such as transferring patients to and from bed, bathing them, and dressing them.)[19] Beyond that, the nurses claimed they did not receive appropriate training to carry out the work, were not paid the promised wage, and were made to care for more patients than is generally accepted as safe. When the nurses left their jobs after exhausting Sentosa's internal-grievance procedures, Sentosa pressed criminal charges for breaking their contracts and sued them for abandoning their patients. It also tried to have the nurses deported. After a two-year battle, the case went to the New York Supreme Court, where in 2010 the charges against the nurses were thrown out, and the nurses were allowed to stay and work in the United States.[20]

Why Hospitals Really Use Staffing Agencies

It's clear that hospitals and nursing homes get workers on the cheap when they hire foreign nurses. But why work through the staffing agencies? The usual stated reason is flexibility: The hospital or nursing home need not commit to hiring a nurse full time. But hospitals and nursing homes already have this flexibility through the use of staff nurses working part-time or overtime.

The real advantage of agency hiring is that it protects the hospital or nursing home from legal liability should the nurse harm a patient. Since the agency, not the hospital, is the nurse's employer, the agency, not the hospital, is ultimately responsible for her performance. If a nurse is highly skilled and adept, the hospital can try to offer her a full-time position. If a nurse is a marginal performer, the hospital can use her on only a temporary basis, when it is short staffed. The tragedy is that the single-year savings of hiring a nurse as staff rather than using an agency nurse are greater than the annual cost of training a nurse in the United States.

Medicare and Medicaid have minimum staffing guidelines for nurse-to-patient ratios for health facilities they reimburse. A hospital with an insufficient number of nurses cannot admit patients, which will cause it to lose money. It can force its staff nurses to work overtime. According to US labor law, clinical nurses are hourly workers, and when they work overtime, they must be compensated at one and a half times their hourly wage. So when a hospital experiences a shortage of nurses, and its staff nurses have maxed out their mandatory overtime, it uses agency nurses. Working for nurse agencies, these nurses are placed in whatever healthcare facility is short of workers.

Hospitals in areas of the country with chronic nurse shortages have had to rely on per-diem, or agency, nurses. This is an expensive way to fill those vacancies, especially when you consider that the average vacancy rate, or percentage of nurses needed, at the nation's hospitals and nursing homes is 8.5 percent. Almost 10 percent!

Even when hospitals hire foreign healthcare workers directly as full-time employees, they can save $40,000 to $50,000 a year. The savings occur on two levels: (1) most foreign-trained nurses are willing to work for less than American nurses; and (2) since the United States does not train enough nurses, the only additional American nurses are temp nurses, who are far more expensive.

A study done by the Washington, DC-based research institute Academy Health revealed that hospitals and nursing homes very consciously view hiring foreign nurses as a way to keep healthcare-worker wages low. These institutions know that in addition to accepting lower wages, foreign healthcare workers demand no signing bonuses or costly continuing education.[21] Moreover, they initially have a higher retention rate than American workers. It takes several years for these workers to learn how to apply for jobs in the United States and to build up their network and professional references, especially if they are working for staffing agencies.

Selling Visas Instead of Training Healthcare Workers

Hospital and healthcare lobbies are among the most powerful in Washington, DC. But whenever Congress places annual caps on the number of visas available for foreign healthcare workers, the hospital lobby pushes for more visas rather than using their political clout to get more American healthcare workers trained and put to work. They do this because, in the short term at least, it is the easiest way to fill healthcare-worker vacancies.

Even the US military has joined in giving US citizenship to foreign healthcare workers. Through the Military Accessions Vital to National Interest program, foreign healthcare workers who enlist in one of the armed services are fast-tracked to citizenship in return for their service.[22] You would think that at the very least the military should train to meet its own vital healthcare needs.

The history of earmarked skill-based visas goes back to the 1920s, when some Americans voiced concern that, in the wake of the devastation wrought by World War I, unskilled Eastern European immigrants were flooding into the country. From there, it was not difficult to see the commercial and military advantage of enticing the most educated workers here, especially with the important role played by foreign scientists during World War II, particularly in developing the atomic bomb. The Hart-Celler Immigrant Act of 1965, which gave preference in immigration to highly skilled people and their families, was the first bill to codify this view.[23]

In 1990, Congress took the act further and created a new category of visa, the H-1B visa, for "temporary workers." These visas, which must be sponsored by an employer, are valid for three years and have an automatic three-year extension. It's not difficult to get further extensions. It may not surprise you to learn that healthcare workers are among the main recipients of the H-1B visa.

Nine years later, Congress passed the Nursing Relief for Disadvantaged Areas Act, which created the H-1C visa, to allow foreign nurses to work in parts of the country that do not have enough nurses. Not surprisingly, access to this visa led to a spike in the number of foreign nurses coming to this country, and relieved the pressure to train more of our own young people to become nurses. When those H-1C visas expired, the number of foreign nurses coming to the United States decreased. It seems clear that the only constraint on foreign healthcare workers entering the United States is the number of visas available, and Congress alone controls this number.

The J-1 visa is one of the major ways by which physicians permanently enter the United States. Yet according to its founding documents, the purpose of the J-1 Exchange Visitor Program is to promote mutual understanding, between the people of the United States and of other countries through temporary educational and cultural exchanges. A State Department website describing the visa says: "Exchange Programs provide an extremely valuable opportunity to experience the US and our way of life, thereby developing lasting and meaningful relationships."[24] The program is run by the US Department of State Office of Private Sector Exchange, the same unit that processes visas for au pairs. The "Private Sector" label for the office is particularly ironic, because most of the physicians using the J-1 visa are leaving public-sector jobs in their home countries.

These are not the only visas available to foreign healthcare workers. Some foreign healthcare workers come here on dependent visas, with a spouse who is entering on a special visa. Some come here through regular visa lotteries, which are not associated with occupation.

And many nurses enter the United States on educational visas. How can this be when educational slots for American nurses are in such short supply? The answer is more short-term thinking. It is very expensive to train a nurse in the United States, and foreign students pay much higher tuition than American students do. Because the schools, too, are only thinking in the short term—and nothing is encouraging them not to—they prefer foreign students because they lose less money on them.

Also, nursing and physical therapy have been declared "Schedule A" shortage occupations. Nurses and physical therapists using this route can access visas without having to go through the individual "certification" of need that is often required in nonhealthcare professions, to prevent employers from importing workers so that they can pay them lower wages.

As I have said before, it is a myth that foreign-trained workers can provide a long-term answer to the healthcare-worker shortage, especially in rural areas of the United States. Within five years of starting a practice in this country, the majority of foreign-trained doctors have moved to big cities and academic areas. Through the J-1 visa-waiver program, in exchange for a green card and a permanent stay in the United States,[25] the federal government tries to entice foreign-trained doctors who have completed their residencies in the United States to practice in rural areas for at least three years. But these physicians have other ways of gaining permanent residency. Since most foreign-trained physicians want to work in major academic centers and metropolitan areas, only about half of the J-1 visa waivers are used. These physicians can find other ways (especially through an H-1B visa or marriage to an American citizen) to stay in the United States.[26]

Foreign-trained nurses, and some doctors, may work in underserved communities, or in healthcare facilities that have a hard time hiring workers because of low pay or undesirable work environment or location. But once foreign-trained nurses have served the obligatory time in their first assignment, they, too, tend to move from the underserved areas to which they have been recruited to major metropolitan areas. The 2000 US Census found that most foreign-born nurses work in California, New York, New Jersey, Florida, and Illinois, states with large metropolitan cities with immigrant communities, not in the states with the greatest nursing shortages: Mississippi, Louisiana, Alabama, and Indiana.[27] Many hospitals report that workers from some countries, particularly the Philippines, will leave the institution as soon as their contracts are up if no large home-country community is in the area.

The majority of foreign healthcare workers are from metropolitan areas in their own countries. They were not and are not attracted by rural life. Not only are foreign healthcare workers recruited through questionable means; they will also never fill the long-term needs of medically underserved communities.

4

The Damage Done

US reliance on foreign healthcare workers hurts not only the health of Americans but that of people in developing countries as well. The negative effects extend in a ripple effect beyond health and cause deleterious social and economic impacts around the world, destabilizing governments and even creating opportunities for terrorist groups. Apart from everything else, global healthcare is a national-security issue.

Lucy, one of our first known human ancestors, lived out her life in a breathtakingly beautiful gorge in the Rift Valley of Ethiopia. Not much is known about Lucy's life. We know that she walked upright, used tools, and had a humanlike pelvis. We don't know what killed Lucy; perhaps she died in childbirth—which would make her very much like her Ethiopian sisters of today. Not a lot of progress in 3.2 million years!

The healthcare-worker shortage is so acute in Ethiopia that only 6 percent of the women have a skilled midwife or doctor to assist them during childbirth. In the United States, where virtually all women have a medical professional present when they give birth, 15 women die of pregnancy-related complications per 100,000 live births. In Ethiopia, 720 women die of pregnancy-related complications per 100,000 live births.[1] More than 99 percent of all maternal deaths occur in developing countries. Almost all of these deaths could be prevented with proper medical assistance.

Nationwide, Ethiopia has an estimated shortage of 10,000 healthcare workers. Much of this shortage can be ascribed to the loss of healthcare workers who emigrated to developed countries. In a 2008 Georgetown University study, a group of recently graduated nurses and physicians in Ethiopia were asked about their career plans. The researchers were amazed to discover that 80 percent of the nurses and 60 percent of the doctors planned to emigrate. Many had already applied for visas.

In 2009, I visited a healthcare clinic in the Rift Valley, Lucy's old stomping grounds. The building was acceptable: It had concrete walls and floors, a sheet-metal roof, a functioning water pump, and a latrine. What it did not have was a doctor or nurse. The staff consisted solely of a sanitarian, whose training was in teaching families about basic hygiene, such as washing hands and how to build a latrine. He was doing what he could, but he had no training in the diagnosis and treatment of disease and only a basic understanding of the medicines and equipment in the clinic. And he was the only healthcare worker for a hundred miles.

Where was the doctor? Most likely in Chicago, where there are more Ethiopian doctors than in all of Ethiopia.

In Ghana, as a study conducted in 2009 for the World Bank showed, 60 percent of the doctors and nurses trained there since it became an independent country, in 1957, have emigrated to the United States or the United Kingdom.[2] Some African countries, despite continually training doctors, have no more physicians now than they did when they attained independence, in the late 1950s or 1960s.

There are more Malawian physicians in Manchester, England, than in Malawi. A small country in the heart of Africa, Malawi has never had a war or a famine, so these doctors are not refugees who fled for their lives. Nor does Britain lack students qualified to enter medical school. It has the professors to teach them and enough world-class institutions in which they can learn. Like the United States, until recently Britain simply found it cheaper to import doctors than to train them.

The Indian doctor is rapidly becoming the face of American medicine, from mind/body guru Dr. Deepak Chopra to medical novelist Dr. Abraham Verghese, from countless Indian doctors on popular television shows to the Indian doctors who practice in your town. Indians make up 25 percent of all foreign-trained doctors in the United States—the largest group of foreign-trained doctors here. So it may surprise you to learn that India has the biggest healthcare-worker deficit of any country in the world.

To the casual observer, it may appear that there are plenty of physicians in India. It has some of the finest hospitals in the world. Indian hospital groups—such as the Apollo Hospital system (not related to the Apollo Group mentioned in chapter 2), with more than 8,500 beds in 50 hospitals throughout India—rival North America and Europe's best medical institutions, with equal or better success rates for complicated procedures, such as heart-bypass surgery. The United Kingdom's National Health Service regularly sends patients to India for faster, more cost-effective care.

Yet this seeming abundance belies the realities. In an address to the Indian Postgraduate Institute of Medical Education and Research in 2009, Indian prime minister Dr. Manmohan Singh observed that "a review of the National Rural Health Mission points out the acute shortage of human resources at various levels. . . . This is one of the biggest impediments to the strengthening of the public-health delivery system and to scaling up access to healthcare."[3]

Because India's healthcare-worker shortage is distributed across a country with the world's second-largest population—

1.18 billion people, or 17 percent of all the people on the planet—its healthcare-worker deficit in terms of total numbers is larger than that in any other country. When you look at rural India—with 860 million residents, 73 percent of the Indian population—you find less than 0.1 healthcare worker per 1,000 residents.[4] The World Health Organization considers India one of the world's 57 health-workforce-crisis countries, because it has fewer than WHO's recommended absolute minimum standard: 2.3 doctors, nurses, and midwives per 1,000 population ("health-worker density").[5]

In order to meet that standard for the most basic health needs, India requires another 456,000 doctors, nurses, midwives, and other healthcare workers—almost half a million. More than 20 countries have a population smaller than India's healthcare-worker deficit! If those 860 million people in rural India made up a nation, it would rank at the absolute bottom in world rankings of health-worker density. This is the country from which the United States imports the largest number of foreign physicians.

Impact on Health

US reliance on importing healthcare workers has a direct negative impact on the health of the people left behind. Studies show that the farther a family lives from a staffed clinic, the more likely its members are to die when they get sick. Traveling to faraway clinics represents a loss of income from missed work, as well as a potential outlay of money for transportation, food, and lodging. Because of the time and expense involved, a family may delay going to a clinic, hoping the family member will get better on his or her own. A study done by WHO in 2005 indicated that in Mali, with every 10 miles a family has to travel for medical care, children's mortality rates rise by 5 percent. A similar study conducted in Burkina Faso demonstrated that after adjusting for confounders such as poverty, child mortality was 50 percent higher for children four hours from a health facility than children with a staffed health facility in their village.[6] The distance from a healthcare worker has a direct effect on life and death.

The United States has 13 doctors, nurses, and midwives for every 1,000 people. Bolivia has 1.05 per 1,000 people; Bangladesh, 0.47; Ethiopia, 0.23. To put it another way, Ethiopia has fewer than five doctors, nurses, and midwives for every 10,000 people in that country. Every WHO study done on the relationship between maternal and child mortality and the number of doctors and nurses per population has found a positive correlation: The larger the number of doctors and nurses per population, the better the health outcomes. This correlation holds regardless of the wealth of a country or its citizens' level of education.

Another study found that health-worker density had a direct correspondence with basic childhood-vaccination coverage, the cornerstone of public health.[7] The countries that had lost the greatest proportion of their healthcare workers to migration were the least able to protect their children from age-old scourges such as polio, pertussis, and tetanus.

In Zambia, for example, a country that has experienced peace since its independence from Britain, in 1964, the infant-mortality rate is 76 per 1,000. That means that of 1,000 children born today, 76 will die before their first birthday. The under-five child-mortality rate in Zambia is 182 per 1,000. That means that almost one in five children born in Zambia dies before his or her fifth birthday.

With the emigration of every nurse and doctor, entire communities—sometimes entire states, with hundreds of thousands of residents—can lose their only healthcare worker. Clearly, these communities are being decimated. The word *decimate* should put this staggering fact into perspective. The word comes from the Roman wartime practice of punishing a losing army by randomly killing one in every 10 of its soldiers. The children in the poorest, most vulnerable communities in the world are being doubly decimated: One in five dies before his or her fifth birthday. How can we in the United States justify the decimation, twice over, of children in the developing world because we do not want to bear the "expense" of training our own children to become doctors and nurses?

One argument for importing healthcare workers is that these workers will return to their own countries able to do more good than they would otherwise. The idea is that nurses and doctors, having mastered all they can in their own countries, will learn better, more cutting-edge medical techniques and take that knowledge home with them. This theory presupposes several things: that the healthcare workers return home, that they will work in their country's healthcare sector, and that the type of medicine they practice will align with the country's needs. But research on foreign healthcare workers in the United States indicates that the vast majority do not return home. Many marry US citizens. Their children become citizens and have no interest in moving to a poor country, let alone one in which they have never lived. While I was at the World Bank, I encountered this phenomenon with the non-American bank staff. When employees retired, they were usually asked where they planned to live. Invariably, they replied that they wanted to move back to Bolivia/Botswana/Bangladesh, but their children and grandchildren were in the United States, so they were "forced" to stay.

Apologists of the current system, who like to think that foreign healthcare workers return home to practice, call this model of immigration "circular migration." But circular migration is a myth, a dream presented to distract people from the reality that nurses and physicians educated with public funds have abandoned the very people who paid for their education.

The healthcare workers who do return home tend to retire or to provide high-end subspecialty care to wealthy people. These are not activities that improve the healthcare system or the overall health of their country.

Then again, the medical knowledge they have acquired abroad is just not applicable at home. The conditions that Americans suffer from are completely different from the most common medical conditions of people in developing countries. The few diseases and conditions they do have in common—injuries and high blood pressure, for instance—are treated with a completely different set of procedures and medications. The top two causes of child death in the United States are accidents and birth defects. The top two killers of children in Nigeria are diarrhea and malaria. The top two killers of adults in the United States are cancer and heart attacks. The top two killers of adults in Nigeria are malaria and childbirth. Exactly what type of knowledge transfer is supposed to occur here?

The health problems and preventable deaths in developing countries are due to a lack of access to any type of healthcare worker—not to a lack of access to a healthcare worker who knows the latest protocols for the most common deadly diseases in the United State. Yes, people suffer from Alzheimer's and die of cancer in Bangladesh, but those diseases are not the ones that kill or cripple the majority of people. These are not the diseases that so damage a population's health that the country's Gross Domestic Product and economic growth are harmed.

Rather than bringing healthcare knowledge home, foreign-born doctors in the United States are more likely to encourage and assist their colleagues to emigrate. Well versed in how the American system works and deeply trusted by their countrymen, they serve as guides to navigating entry into the American clinical system. Some foreign-born healthcare workers have organized diaspora groups by country of origin, most notably the American Association of Physicians of Indian Origin, Association of Pakistani Physicians of North America, Ghanaian Physicians and Surgeons Foundation of North America, and the Ethiopian North American Health Professionals Association. Their activities tend to advance the careers of their members in the United States or focus on bringing unsustainable, inappropriate technology to their home countries.

Some of these organizations run medical missions, bringing a team of healthcare workers into the home country for a few weeks. But the results of these missions are not sustainable, and the techniques they teach, such as kidney transplants or open-heart surgery, are not the most effective investments in saving lives in those countries—where the major killers are diarrhea, pneumonia, malaria, and vaccine-preventable diseases—and the real problem is lack of access to healthcare workers with even the most basic skills.

These programs divert limited resources from areas in which they can be most cost-effective and save the largest numbers of lives to unsustainable programs whose limited health impact is confined mainly to the wealthy. I have heard deans of medical schools in Africa call for more programs to teach kidney-transplant surgery. If these deans really cared about kidney disease in Africa, they would call for a renewed focus on schistosomiasis, a tropical disease in which centimeter-long worms live in the kidneys and urinary tract, causing suffering, disability, and death. This disease affects 200 million people in Africa. It is treated with a single dose of medicine, but a health worker has to be there to diagnose the disease and administer the medicine.

When my World Bank team hosted a meeting on training

healthcare workers in developing countries, we talked about the need to train healthcare workers appropriate to the needs of the population, such as midwives. A member of the Ghanaian parliament stood up from the audience and denounced the discussion, declaring that none of the Westerners in the room would want a family member to have her delivery attended by a midwife instead of an obstetrician. Why should Ghanaians settle for less? An awkward silence followed as we thought about how to politely inform him that, while obstetricians attend the majority of births in the United States, the majority of births in Europe—which has lower maternal-mortality rates than the United States—are attended by midwives. The Netherlands has invested so heavily in training midwives that most Dutch women deliver in their own homes with a midwife in attendance. Finally, a fellow African delivered the news to the surprised politician.

It just doesn't make sense for an Indian, Kenyan, or Ethiopian physician to train in the United States. The majority of preventable and unnecessary deaths that occur in developing countries—from malaria, dengue fever, severe undernutrition—either are not found in the United States or are extremely rare. The foreign-born physician is better off continuing to practice and hone her skills in her own country. Even if a migrant healthcare worker learns some treatments for a disease prevalent in her country, such as HIV/AIDS or diarrhea, the treatments and methods are irrelevant, because they involve technology and medicines that either are not available in her country or are too expensive.

For example, severe diarrhea, one of the biggest killers of children in developing countries, is treated in the United States with intravenous fluids. In developing countries, the most cost-effective and sustainable way to treat severe diarrhea is through oral rehydration: frequent spoon feeding of specially prepared formulas. If IV fluids are available, they are so expensive that their use needlessly consumes limited resources. Healthcare workers who do return home are often frustrated and discouraged because they cannot practice what they have learned. But sometimes they encourage the use of expensive techniques, which can needlessly reduce the funding available for patients with illnesses that are relatively inexpensive to treat.

Healthcare workers trained outside a country's own healthcare system can actually damage that system, even in a developing county. This phenomenon is evident in the small African country of Lesotho. The country has no medical school, so the government sends students to train in nearby South Africa, the wealthiest country in sub-Saharan Africa. Here, the Lesotho medical students learn about diseases, drugs, techniques, and equipment that are totally irrelevant to saving lives in their own country—cancer chemotherapy protocols, for instance, that include drugs not available in Lesotho, and surgical techniques dependent on equipment such as surgical staples or endoscopes, which are not readily available.

Not surprisingly, few of these students return to Lesotho after graduation. Those who do go home flock to the one tertiary (subspecialty) hospital, the Queen Elizabeth II Hospital, in the capital city of Maseru, where they continue to practice what they learned in South Africa to treat cancer and heart attacks. But in Lesotho, the main cause of death in children is diarrhea and vaccine-preventable illnesses; maternal mortality is on the rise; and only 41 percent of women have access to modern forms of family planning.[8]

At last measure, the Queen Elizabeth II Hospital—a single hospital—consumed 21 percent of the entire budget for the Lesotho Ministry of Health.[9]

Clearly, the strategy of educating physicians in a wealthier country has backfired. It has not improved the health of the people of Lesotho; it has hurt it.

Impact on Health-Education Institutions

Medical and nursing schools in developing countries have been profoundly affected by the fact that the US healthcare market—the largest healthcare market in the world—is so reliant on foreign-trained healthcare workers. In African medical schools, emigration is the number one reason for the loss of professors. And a lack of professors, of course, makes it even more difficult to train the healthcare providers these countries so desperately need. The shortage of professors became so dire in Malawi that the Ministry of Health started to send its staff to the health-professional schools to teach. Not only are we stealing the water; we are also smashing the pump.

Our reliance on foreign healthcare workers is causing other significant problems in health-professional schools in developing countries. For one thing, it is creating a general orientation in healthcare schools toward the needs of the United States and away from those of the home country. In many developing countries, the quality of the medical and nursing schools is informally measured by the ability of the graduates to pass US licensing exams. The alumni practicing in the United States, who see the American system as the gold standard of healthcare education and delivery, have a profound impact on the thinking of the schools' leadership. To facilitate their graduates' entry into the US market, several medical schools in developing countries have even changed their curriculum to match that of American schools.[10]

Many leaders of the healthcare systems in developing countries privately express the hope that extended-family members who are healthcare workers will be able to move to a developed country. That notion gives these leaders a strong incentive to switch the country's health-professional schools to a US-oriented curriculum and give the school a reputation that facilitates the migration. The constant flow of the best and brightest to the United States creates a "culture of leaving," in which it is expected that high achievers will emigrate, and moving to the United States or Europe becomes the best and fastest way to prove one's prowess as a clinician.[11] Students who stay in their own countries—either by choice or because they were unable to pass US licensing exams—are viewed as inferior or backward and parochial.

The net effect is a mismatch between how healthcare workers are trained and the needs and practice realities in their countries—an education system oriented around American health needs rather than local ones. Since most healthcare-worker training in developing countries is paid for with public funds, this situation represents the capture of public money for the private, external gain of individuals rather than for the improvement of national healthcare training and public health.

Some may argue that if the orientation toward American training occurs in private medical or nursing schools, it is of less concern because the resources used are private. This notion is partly true but needs careful scrutiny. In work I conducted with Dr. Alex Preker at the World Bank, we found that even when ownership is private, there is often significant public financing. This occurs in a variety of forms, including scholarships for students; government grants or subsidized loans for investing in infrastructure, such as new buildings; privileged access to public hospitals and clinics for clinical training; and donations of equipment, such as anatomical models or ultrasound machines, channeled through the government.

The problem of foreign health-professional schools oriented toward this country's health needs is about to become even worse. The US Education Commission for Foreign Medical Graduates (ECFMG), the body that certifies foreign-trained physicians to practice in the United States, has traditionally relied solely on evaluations of the individual physicians to determine eligibility. But in September 2010, as the implications of US healthcare reform became more apparent—specifically, that US demands for foreign-trained healthcare workers would only increase—the ECFMG announced that it would begin requiring schools from which foreign-trained physicians had graduated to be "accredited through a formal process that uses criteria comparable to those established for US medical schools by the Liaison Committee on Medical Education."[12]

Now it will not be enough for a school to be accredited by the government of the country in which it is based. There will be incredible pressure for the school to be accredited to US standards by the Liaison Committee on Medical Education or global standards by the World Federation for Medical Education. Most foreign medical schools are already accredited by a national organization composed of local stakeholders, who are aware of local needs and practices. US demand for external accreditation, and the following demand from alumni in the United States and the home country, as well as from current and future students, will undoubtedly distract these leaders from local needs. There is no doubt that the accrediting requirement from the world's largest importer of healthcare workers will lead many medical schools to seek external accreditation and shift their goals.

South Africa provides a clear example of how international accreditation can lead to increased emigration. Because of the United Kingdom's recent history of heavy reliance on foreign medical graduates, the National Health Service accredits medical schools in Britain's former colonies. All of the medical schools in South Africa have chosen to receive this accreditation except for one: Walter Sisulu Medical College, a community-based medical school with a strong commitment to training physicians for the underserved rural Transkei region. Since this school's mission is to train physicians for South Africa rather than for the United Kingdom, it has chosen to be accredited by only the Health Professions Council of South Africa. Because of its strategic choice not to adopt the accreditation standards of other countries, Walter Sisulu Medical School is the *only* medical school in South Africa to have the majority of its graduates practicing in South Africa. The majority of these doctors practice in underserved, rural areas.

Conversely, the internationally accredited South African medical schools—that is to say, all the others—have seen the majority of their graduates leave the country. Why wouldn't they? With a degree from a UK-accredited medical school, they do not need to undergo any additional testing or certification to have their degrees and licenses accepted by the National Health Service. They can land at Heathrow and see patients the next day! The ECFMG's decision to require international accreditation of medical schools will surely facilitate similar large-scale migrations of physicians from the developing world.

Impact on Society

Until recently, a medical doctorate was one of the few advanced degrees available in many African countries. Indeed, in most developing countries, the people with the most education are physicians. It is not surprising that many physicians have become president of their country. Chile's former president, Michelle Bachelet, is a pediatrician. Nepal's president, Ram Baran Yadav, is a physician. Even everyone's favorite revolutionary, Che Guevara, was a physician. Seeing poor people die of easily preventable and curable diseases motivated him to become politically active.

In developing countries, healthcare workers are more than the backbone of the healthcare system; they are the backbone of society. Throughout the developing world, physicians and nurses are active in political parties; they are the key businesspeople and investors; they are deacons of their churches; they support cultural institutions and nongovernmental organizations (NGOS). When importing foreign physicians and nurses, the system selects for those with the most skills, wealth, and connections—those whom the developing countries can least afford to lose. Their loss does far more than damage healthcare in that country. It leaves an unfillable vacuum throughout the length and breadth of society. Imagine the negative impact on your community if every year the 10 smartest, most creative, and most highly motivated people you knew left the country, never to return.

Many people like to think that the United States and other wealthy countries are doing developing countries a favor by employing their health workers. True, many developing countries have terrible unemployment and underemployment problems, as well as much informal employment, wherein no salary is guaranteed.[13] But these unemployed workers tend not to be healthcare workers. Unemployment is a problem among large populations of rural and urban poor, most of whom have only a few years of formal education. In many countries, the majority of people in rural communities are subsistence farmers, who are able to produce little more than what their family needs to eat and who have few opportunities for formal employment.

Healthcare-worker unemployment is relatively rare, and it is usually not unemployed healthcare workers who emigrate. US hospitals will preferentially hire an employed doctor over an unemployed doctor, on the assumption that the worker who has a job is a better performer. The higher the perceived quality of healthcare workers, and the more experience they have, the more likely they are to get licensed and hired in the United States.

Some people justify the importing of foreign healthcare workers because of the money, or "remittances," they send home. Indeed, the total remittance from all migrant workers (not just healthcare workers) is far greater than the total amount of development assistance rich countries give to poor countries each year. The evidence shows that, while the money sent by low-income laborers may be of great help to their families, money sent by high-income workers (such as healthcare workers) has no significant impact on development in the home country.

Why is that? On most types of US earmarked "health" visas, the workers are able to bring their families with them, so there is no need to send money to them. By contrast, undocumented immigrants, especially from Latin America, often leave wives and children at home because illegally crossing the border is both physically arduous and dangerous. When they find work in this country, these workers send relatively large amounts of money to their immediate families, helping to lift them out of poverty.

What about sending money to the extended families of foreign healthcare workers? The extended families usually are well off by local standards; what money is sent to them tends to be spent on luxury items, not on investments such as education and permanent housing. Moreover, most remittances are sent informally rather than through formal banking channels, so this money is not taxed. The home government can recoup none of the cost of training the healthcare worker even in that indirect way.

The flip side of remittances is the cost to the economy from the loss of these highly educated workers. A team of researchers from the WHO Africa bureau calculated that a single physician who leaves Kenya results in a loss of about US $517,931 in returns from the investment in his or her education. The loss to the Kenyan economy from an emigrating nurse is $338,868 in returns on investment.[14]

A similar study in Malawi revealed that when a physician left to work abroad, it created a loss of $433,493 to the Malawian economy over the years of his career. If you use Malawian banking rates of return (25 percent annually) in the calculations, that investment loss skyrockets to $46 million over the physician's career.[15]

Importing healthcare workers is more damaging to source countries than importing other types of workers is. For example, every year the United States imports thousands of highly skilled information technology (IT) workers, such as computer programmers, from India, yet you hear no complaint from India. IT workers cost much less to train and are trained much faster than physicians and nurses, so there is no shortage of them in India, and the financial loss to India of each such emigrant is much lower. More important, no one dies because an IT worker has left a community.

When most Americans think of immigrant labor, they think of the 9 million undocumented and 12 million legal Latino immigrants in the United States.[16] But this migrant labor force could not be more different from the migrant healthcare labor force, in both its composition and its effects on their home countries. On arrival in the United States, many Latino immigrants have no high school education, know little or no English, and are functionally illiterate in their native Spanish. Immigrant healthcare workers tend to know English and have bachelor's or higher-level degrees from the most elite universities in their countries. The average Latino migrant leaves home because he or she has no job, or has a job that does not feed the family or that offers little advancement. Foreign healthcare workers leave government jobs with salaries that put them in the top 10 percent of earners in their country—jobs with pensions, health and housing benefits, and virtual tenure.

For many Latin American countries, US immigration is a stabilizing force, a sort of release valve for social tensions. For example, the emigration of hundreds of thousands of El Salvadorans to the United States in the 1980s, during El Salvador's civil war, served as an outlet for political opponents of the government. For Latin American countries without active conflicts, the emigration of the rural poor relieves the social pressure that might build up if large numbers of the poor and unemployed organized into a mass movement. Losing uneducated citizens is not considered damaging to these countries, because they have invested little or nothing in them: no education, no social services. In fact, these countries benefit from the remittances migrant laborers send home. Remittances from nonhealthcare workers are often the number one or number two source of foreign currency in Latin American countries.

These realities explain why the governments of many Latin American countries turn a blind eye to unskilled emigration, while those of Caribbean, African, and Asian countries officially protest the loss of their highly skilled healthcare workers.

Impact on US Minorities and Their Communities

In this country, the biggest losers from our dependence on foreign-born healthcare workers are minority students and communities. Latinos and African Americans are grossly underrepresented among healthcare workers: They make up 27 percent of the US population but only 10 percent of US nurses and physicians. Because these minority communities tend to be the most medically underserved, it is these communities that are cited as justification for importing foreign healthcare workers. We rely on foreign-trained healthcare workers to serve minority communities rather than training young people from those communities to become healthcare workers.

African Americans and Latinos often have few or no members of their family who have graduated from college; they tend to have even fewer role models in the medical and nursing fields. Many Latino students considering a career in healthcare may be the first member of their family to graduate from high school. Also, African American and Latino students often graduate from poorer-quality high schools and second-tier colleges. This makes their medical and nursing applications less competitive than those from white and Asian American students, who are more likely to have attended high-performing high schools and top-tier colleges. Even the best African American and Latino students may not have had the opportunities to ornament their résumés in the way their white and Asian American peers of equal ability have.

Our system of financing medical and nursing education requires students to take on huge sums of education debt. The American Medical Association estimates that the average medical student graduates with $156,000 in debt. Multiple studies have shown that as education debt increases, more people from underserved communities choose not to attend medical school. Those who do attend are more likely to pursue specialty practices in higher-paying metropolitan areas rather than the more needed primary care in underserved communities.

So, not surprisingly, financing is one of the main reasons that Latinos and African Americans have found it difficult to enter medical and nursing schools in large numbers. According to the

US Census Bureau, the average income of African American families is 30 percent lower than that of white families. This discourages many potential students from minority families from going to college, let alone to medical or nursing school. And many African American and Latino families have little or no experience with loans of any type, whether student loans or even home mortgages. This lack of understanding of and comfort with loans makes minority students less likely to pursue careers that necessitate taking out large student loans.

Minority families' lower incomes force those who do pursue higher education to either work at the same time, which diminishes their focus on their studies, or rely more on student loans. On average, minority students who graduate from either college or medical or nursing school do so with a higher burden of debt than white students. A number of research studies have shown that concerns about paying off student debt are a barrier for African Americans and Latinos considering medical or nursing careers.[17]

Although minorities are underrepresented among nurses and physicians, they are overrepresented in lower-level healthcare positions, such as nursing assistants, lab technicians, and phlebotomists, who specialize in drawing blood. The large numbers of minorities in lower-level positions surely reflects the desire of minorities to work in the healthcare field. The discrepancy between their numbers in low-level and high-level positions reflects what I call the "gauze ceiling," which prevents minorities from accessing higher-level healthcare training. The gauze ceiling represents an opportunity for the United States to mend both educational and healthcare-access wrongs. Special programs to facilitate the entry of minorities into health-professional schools would help tear down the gauze ceiling and allow minority communities eventually to gain more access to healthcare workers.

Importing healthcare workers is not the answer to meeting the needs of underserved populations in this country. The best solution is to train healthcare workers within these communities. In 1989, when the population of New York State was 20 percent African American and Latino, just 8 percent of the practicing physicians were African American or Latino. Then the 14 medical schools in that state started a high school–based program to increase interest among African American and Latino students in careers in medicine. Now those schools are graduating minorities in numbers equivalent to their share of the population. Not only has this improved these communities' access to health workers; it has improved their economies as well.

Studies on the patient populations and practice areas of minority nurses and doctors indicate that these workers are more likely than whites to practice in minority areas and to serve minority patients. In fact, studies from all over the world demonstrate that the best strategy for placing and retaining healthcare providers in underserved communities is to train people from those communities. This finding is significant, because the death and disability disparities between these patients and white patients are huge. On average, African Americans die a full decade earlier than whites; Latinos have five times the rate of diabetes and twice the obesity rates of whites.

Imported healthcare workers may practice in underserved minority areas for a few years, until they gain permanent residency. But as soon as they achieve citizenship or a green card, they actually are less likely than US-born clinicians to practice in underserved and rural areas, and are more likely to be found in academic centers and wealthy cities. This phenomenon reflects the workers' primary motivations for leaving home in the first place: education and career opportunities and increased compensation—advantages found to a much greater extent in metropolitan areas.

In addition, while most imported healthcare workers are not white, they are not from the cultures of the American minorities with the greatest healthcare needs. Africans are not African Americans. In many US cities with large African communities, tensions have arisen with the local African American communities over issues such as values, jobs, culture, and crime. In Washington, DC, problems between the Ethiopian and African American communities have required mediation by city councillors. Other cultures that are overrepresented among immigrant healthcare workers include Indians and Filipinos, whose communities in the United States are neither poor nor medically underserved.

What about healthcare workers from Latin America? Despite the infusion of healthcare workers from Latin American countries, their total number is insufficient to meet the needs of the Latino community in the United States. More important, this community is not monolithic. It includes Mexicans, El Salvadorans, Cubans, Puerto Ricans, Dominicans, Peruvians, and a dozen others—each community with its own rich traditional medicine and unique cultural take on health, illness, and patient-healer relationships.

Impact on US Security

High rates of poor health and premature death can destabilize a country. This is even more true with potential or actual epidemic diseases—HIV/AIDS, SARS, avian flu, dengue fever, malaria, and dozens more—which can quickly break down the structure of society by causing schools and workplaces to close and overwhelming social-support systems. As rapid transport has made the world "smaller," multi-drug-resistant tuberculosis and diseases with 90 percent mortality rates, such as Ebola and Marburg, are only a plane ride away. Beyond that, weak, destabilized countries can give rise to homegrown political insurgencies and terrorist groups whose actions can affect this country.

In the 1980s, the devastation of HIV/AIDS raised the world's awareness of the national-security risks that health crises in poor countries can pose to developed countries. In January 2000, the United Nations Security Council held its first-ever meeting focused on a health issue—that is, on HIV/AIDS. Declaring AIDS "a global aggressor that must be defeated," then-vice president Al Gore blamed Africa's challenges in addressing AIDS on its "weak infrastructure."[18] A big part of that weak infrastructure was the lack of leaders to run the countries' healthcare systems; another was having too few physicians, nurses, and other healthcare providers in place or being trained to provide the treatment and lessons in prevention needed to control and stop the epidemic. That year, the Security Council adopted Resolution 1308, which recognized the role of HIV/AIDS and of a population's health in general in peacekeeping and security.

From there, it was a quick step to the recognition that almost any disease, if unchecked, could threaten our own security. The issue is so important that both the Bush and Obama administrations included health in their national-security strategies. The United States made the world's largest investment in addressing the global HIV/AIDS crisis in the current $48 billion President's Emergency Plan for AIDS Relief. According to former President George W. Bush, "during a presidency often forced to focus on issues of national security, the fight against global disease was sometimes viewed as an anomaly or exception. It wasn't and isn't. America has a direct stake in the progress and hope of other nations."[19] The Obama national-security strategy notes that the United States "has a moral and strategic interest in promoting global health. When a child dies of a preventable disease, it offends our conscience; when a disease goes unchecked, it can endanger our own health; when children are sick, development is stalled."[20]

Reflecting this thinking on the links between health in developing countries and our own security, the US military has set up an entire program centered on global health. This program provides healthcare directly to areas with little home-government capacity and assists governments in disaster response. An excellent example is the US military's response to the Haitian earthquake, in early 2010. The medical care provided by the military hospital ship *Comfort* and many US military-led clinics helped prevent a fragile postdisaster situation from becoming even more unstable.[21]

If the government of a country cannot provide basic health services, sometimes other, less democratic forces will. In the Palestinian territories, Hamas was able to provide basic healthcare for communities in which the Fatah-led government was not doing so. Hamas's main path to legitimacy and political support was its effective provision of healthcare and social services.[22] Providing these services was a major reason that Hamas defeated the PLO-affiliated Fatah in the 2006 elections to the Palestinian parliament. Similarly, other terrorist or criminal groups, such as the Taliban in areas of Afghanistan and neighborhood-based drug gangs in Jamaica, have won hearts and minds by providing healthcare services when the legitimate government does not.

In a 2009 report on global health and US security, the Center for Strategic International Studies, in Washington, DC, recommended "putting a high priority on meeting the health needs of developing countries as core elements of a U.S. strategy to address the national-security threats of emerging infectious diseases and bioterrorism."[23]

Unfortunately, those in charge of national security and the

hundreds of people and organizations controlling our underproduction of healthcare workers do not communicate with each other. Worse, they seem unaware that their actions and policies are at cross-purposes. As mentioned earlier, the US military is an active participant in the importing of health workers.

In January 2009, the US Institute of Medicine and the US Africa Command, the division of the Department of Defense responsible for all US military operations in Africa, held a symposium on "Health as a Bridge to Peace and Stability." The purpose was to introduce the Africa Command's new chief surgeon, Colonel Dr. Schuyler K. Geller, to potential healthcare partners within and outside the US government. The symposium marked a huge step in recognizing and acting on the links between US national-security interests and health, in Africa as well as in other regions with poor health statistics.

Yet not one person with responsibilities for domestic production of healthcare workers attended. Not a single person who could have worked with the US military to stop our unintentional destabilization of developing countries—which is what we do by recruiting their best healthcare workers—was there.

The Fox and the Hydra

Failed Attempts to Address Insourcing

The origin of the healthcare-worker shortage can be traced to two unfortunate elements of the national and global healthcare markets, which I call the fox and the Hydra. The proverbial foxes guarding the henhouse are the health-professional organizations that limit the number of workers in their fields, unnecessarily drive up the cost of their education, and create a mismatch between what health workers learn and what they need for their jobs. The Hydra, the Greek mythical creature with seven heads (which grew two for every one that was cut off), is an uncoordinated regulatory system, with national and international players operating independently of one another and using short-term solutions that have actually increased insourcing.

Management of the healthcare workforce, in the United States and abroad, has evolved from an essentially free-market system to one that combines the worst aspects of the free market and regulation. Uncoordinated central authorities control the production of healthcare workers, and the free market allows them to move across national and international borders regardless of their legal commitments or where they are needed most. You might call this broken system "uncoordinated regulation."

A true free market for healthcare-worker education and employment would look something like this: Schools for doctors, nurses, physical therapists, and other healthcare providers, which would open and close at will, would be free to train as many students as were willing to pay for an education. Competition among the schools would drive down costs while maintaining quality. The graduates would work wherever they found patients who could pay for their services or hospitals willing to employ them. Schools that trained substandard practitioners, unable to find jobs or sufficient patients because of the school's poor reputation, would eventually close. Conversely, schools with reputations for high-quality programs and graduates would expand and open new branches, as paying students flocked to them.

A true regulated system would look like this: Some central authority, either government or private, would oversee education and employment and would ensure adequate numbers, quality, and distribution of healthcare workers. This authority would open and close schools, decide how many students each would train, and incentivize where the graduates worked. Schools deemed to produce substandard graduates would either receive sufficient guidance to improve or be shut down. Schools producing superior graduates would expand, and schools performing less well would learn the better schools' training methods.

In a free-market system, no one is looking at the system as a whole; the individual schools, students, healthcare workers, and employers make decisions independently to benefit themselves. No one tries to address any gaps in the system, which tend to be filled via supply and demand. The thinking is that if a region doesn't have enough healthcare workers, entrepreneurs will open schools to meet the demand, and employers and patients will pay more, drawing both students and healthcare workers to that region.

In a central-authority system, the authority monitors the system as a whole. If that authority determines there aren't enough healthcare workers in a region, it opens new schools and creates incentives for healthcare workers to move there.

In the ideal free-market and central-authority systems, shortages are resolved and quality is kept high. Unfortunately, ideal worlds rarely exist. In the real world of healthcare, both systems are deeply flawed.

Why the Free-Market System Failed: Flexner and the AMA

In the early 1900s, there were few healthcare workers other than nurses and physicians. Nursing skills revolved mainly around administering oral medications, feeding, and bathing, so the quality of care depended less on the education and more on the motivation of the individual nurse. Nurses were trained in hospitals, and because they generally found work in the same hospital, their employers were well aware of their level of skill.

As for medical schools, most of them were "proprietary," meaning they were private schools owned by one or two physicians and run for a profit. The faculty tended to be physicians who practiced in the community; the students, too, were from that community. With few if any regulations, it was fairly easy to open a medical school. If the school developed a poor reputation and students stopped seeking it out, the school would shut down. Because there were very few state-funded schools, few bad schools were propped up with state funds. But the length of training, the content of the training, and the amount of clinical experience students received at the schools varied greatly.

This is the setting in which the American Medical Association asked the Carnegie Foundation to fund the nationwide study of medical education that I described in chapter 2. Published in 1910, the Flexner Report (the official title is *Medical Education in the United States and Canada*) became one of the most important publications on its topic in the world. The problem was that Abraham Flexner, who was not a doctor, chose to focus his study very narrowly. In his model of public health, conveying knowledge of the latest scientific advances was the main criteria for a good medical education. In that regard, the small, more rural proprietary schools lagged behind the larger, mainly metropolitan, university- and hospital-based schools. What Flexner failed to realize is that the number and accessibility of health workers and the relevance of their education is just as important as the quality of their care. A well-trained doctor that lives and practices in your home town and has skills relevant to your care is more likely to make a difference in your health than a superbly trained research doctor locked away in an ivory tower.

The Flexner Report had a dramatic negative effect on the physician workforce. The local medical schools had easily adjusted class sizes to meet local needs, but the big state schools that replaced them rarely varied their output of students. These students tended to be from elite families in the big cities in which the schools were based and rarely left those cities to practice. Since the physicians from the proprietary schools were from the communities they served, they cared for their neighbors and friends regardless of ability to pay.[1] The physicians trained in the large metropolitan schools did not follow this practice, thus shutting the poor out of access to medical care.

Another effect of the report, as noted in chapter 2, was the plummeting enrollment of women and African Americans, diminishing the access of women and minority communities to medical care.[2] The number of physicians per capita dropped in many regions and leveled off nationally.

The shortage of primary-care physicians also began with the consolidation of medical education at the university level. When physicians were trained in small, local schools, they usually entered primary care. In the university setting, where research and subspecialties tend to be seen as more important than primary care, more and more physicians chose to subspecialize.

As noted earlier, the Flexner Report resulted in the consolidation or closing of more than half the medical schools in the country. In the early 1900s, there were around 160 medical schools at a time when the population was 76 million (so: one medical school per half million people). By 1920, that number had fallen to 85 medical schools. By 1935, there were only 66 medical schools in the country. Today we're almost back to where we were in the early 1900s. The United States currently has 161 medical schools (133 MD-granting schools and 28 DO-granting schools). But the country's population is now 310 million, so the current ratio is one medical school per every 2 million people.

The reason so many schools closed once the Flexner Report came out was that rather than trying to improve the poorer-performing schools, the AMA chose to shut them down. Essentially a physicians' guild, it became the de facto regulator of medical schools in the United States. The federal government might have had a broader interest in ensuring access to healthcare, but surprisingly, the Department of Health and Human Services was a very late entrant into the health sector. There was no cabinet-level health post until 1953, when President Eisenhower established the Department of Health, Education, and Welfare. There was no office focused solely on healthcare issues until 1980, when President Carter established an independent Department of Health and Human Services. With the federal government essentially uninvolved in the healthcare workforce, the AMA established a pattern of uncoordinated, guild-led regulation, and the other healthcare professionals—nurses, pharmacists, dentists, podiatrists, optometrists, physical therapists, occupational therapists, and dozens of others—developed similar means of self-regulation.

World War II and "Manpower Planning"

After 1910, guild-led regulation and the notions put forth in the Flexner Report became the predominant model of healthcare-worker education in the United States, Europe, and, by extension to their colonies in Africa, Asia, and Latin America, throughout the rest of the world. Then came World War II, which caused a sea change in attitudes toward coordinated planning. The combatant states devoted more than half of their national output and two-thirds of their industrial workforce to wartime production.[3] With coordinated planning, agricultural and industrial outputs increased substantially. The education of healthcare workers was ramped up, too; this included a temporary doubling of the annual production of physicians in the US.

Tens of thousands of Allied and Axis citizens serving in the military were exposed to scientific management and planning.[4] After the war, millions of people on both sides began to apply newly learned scientific-management skills to civilian activities. At the same time, the Soviet Union arose as an economic, political, and military powerhouse, exerting particular influence in Africa and parts of Asia. These military and Soviet influences propelled "manpower planning" and "manpower studies,"[5] which examined how many of what types of workers were needed and advised industries on production numbers. In the United States, the Department of Labor funded manpower centers to perform these assessments and provide technical assistance in all fields.

The postwar period of the 1950s and 1960s represented the

heyday of coordinated healthcare-workforce planning. Most European countries had central-planning boards responsible for looking past guild interests to the workforce needs of the healthcare system as a whole. With its health-manpower centers, the United States, too, studied trends in healthcare-worker production, productivity, and demand.

It was during this time that some of the most rational steps were taken to ensure that all Americans, no matter where they lived or how much they earned, had access to qualified healthcare workers. In 1965 Medicare made health insurance available to millions of previously uninsured Americans, which, of course, increased the need for healthcare workers. A year later, Congress passed the Allied Health Professions Personnel Act (PL-751), promoting the development of programs to train new types of primary-care providers. Physician assistants and nurse practitioners, both envisioned as more cost-effective ways of delivering primary healthcare to poor and rural communities, can trace their professional origins to the Allied Health Professions Personnel Act. These changes led to a general increase in the supply of healthcare workers.

Until World War II, most of the healthcare workers in both the United States and Europe had studied in private, nonstate schools. Now, under the military- and Soviet-influenced systems, governments began producing these workers in public schools and dictating their types and numbers. Many newly independent countries founded their first medical and nursing schools following this model. For decades, these public schools used their influence to keep competing private schools from opening.

Around the world, the presumption of these newly formed public schools was that all graduates would go into public-sector jobs or would open practices where the need was greatest. No attention was paid to the geographic regions from which the students came—and, just as with the free-market approach, the vast majority of students came from metropolitan areas. These students, too, chose to stay near their families and refused jobs in rural or underserved areas. Because the national systems paid specialists more, the majority of graduates went into specialty care.

The central-planning approach was government focused, and thus blind to the private sector and to the choices of individuals. In addition, it looked only at the total numbers of healthcare workers, not at their geographic or specialty distribution. Worse, the assumption was that the per capita need for healthcare workers would remain constant, rather than grow as technology, family incomes, and healthcare funding increased. By the end of the 1970s, many countries erroneously believed they were meeting or even exceeding their needs for healthcare workers. In the 1980s, different groups with a variety of assumptions regarding healthcare-worker supply and demand began predicting an *oversupply* of healthcare workers. The United States predicted a physician surplus.

Despite gross inequalities in the distribution of healthcare workers, countries everywhere capped their production of these workers. For decades, even as the global population grew rapidly, the total numbers of healthcare workers stayed flat. In the United States and elsewhere, almost all healthcare-workforce planning ceased. Within five years after the US withdrawal from central planning, not a single Western European country had a healthcare-workforce planning unit.[6]

Back to the Free-Market Approach

As the failures of the Soviet system and the problems in managing the healthcare workforce through central planning became obvious, the world moved back to more of a free-market approach. Believing the market would determine how many healthcare workers were needed and where, governments greatly reduced or halted the collection of data in those areas.

For free markets to function effectively, though, they must be free from overregulation. In the 1980s and '90s, overregulation came from a surprising source: the healthcare-worker associations themselves. All around the world, the boards, committees, and institutions that governed licensing for healthcare workers and schools put up barriers to growth. Fearful of competition and loss of income, the professional guilds tightly regulated membership, restricting their numbers via school-enrollment caps and increased licensure requirements.

These organizations stymied the production of what they saw as competing healthcare professionals, such as nurse practitioners and auxiliary nurses. The ostensible reason for, say, raising the number of years of training required to practice was always to improve quality; but the resultant lack of access to healthcare workers actually worsened health outcomes. With their numbers capped or declining and the freedom to move wherever they liked, healthcare workers regionally and globally once again concentrated in metropolitan areas. Again, laissez-faire achieved the economic goal of distributing a limited resource to those who had the most money, but offered no free-market means of producing more.

During this period, most countries conducted virtually no coordinated management or planning of their national healthcare workforces. For the most part, the field of healthcare-workforce management remained dormant.

As for wealthier countries aiding the healthcare-workforce efforts of developing countries, the focus was mainly on short-term programs to increase quality of care—that is, on retraining healthcare workers rather than on training new ones.

This well-meaning practice was based on two misconceptions. The first is that preventable deaths in developing countries are due to a lack of knowledge—that most such deaths occur because the healthcare worker doesn't know what is wrong with the patient or what can be done to save him or her. Nothing could be further from the truth. In developing countries, the vast majority of people who die unnecessarily are infants, children, and pregnant women who die in their own homes, having never been seen by a healthcare worker because none is available. If they do manage to get help, it is frequently too late; the patients are too ill for anything to be done for them. However, if a patient can get to a healthcare worker in a timely manner, the healthcare provider usually can make a difference.

Often, however—because the healthcare system is poorly run, the leaders and managers having been recruited to other countries—the drugs or equipment to treat the patient are lacking. This problem reflects an important phenomenon known as the know/do gap: the difference between what a healthcare worker knows (as measured by a test) and what a healthcare worker does (as measured by observation or interviews with patients). In developing countries in Africa and Asia, in public and private hospitals and clinics, researchers consistently have found a wide gap between what healthcare workers know and what they are able to do for patients. More training just increases that gap, as well as healthcare workers' frustration over their inability to use their knowledge and skills.

The second misconception is that if a donor country pays to create more health-professional schools, the developing country may not have the resources to maintain them or to hire the new graduates. The evidence belies this. In developing countries, healthcare workers have virtually guaranteed employment for life, at salaries in the upper 10 or 20 percent, and extended families are willing and able to pay for the education of family members. In fact, a recent study found that the most rapid growth in medical schools in Africa was in private medical schools, where students paid out of pocket for the full cost of their education.[7] Financial sustainability is not an issue in training healthcare workers in the developing world.

As for employing new healthcare workers, most developing countries have double-digit healthcare-worker vacancy rates, with hundreds or thousands of budgeted-for positions that they cannot find anyone to fill. Private practices and private hospitals in developing countries are also experiencing staff shortages.

Focusing on the short-term training of existing workers is attractive to donor governments because it is easily accomplished and shows fast "results." It does not cost much to fly trainers in to a capital city for a few weeks. Healthcare workers are paid a per diem to attend the training sessions, so attendance rates are high, and project managers can report on the number of workers whose skills have been upgraded. Rarely, however, is there any follow-up to see whether the workers are using their new skills or whether the training has led to a decrease in deaths. Indeed, it is quite common to hear about healthcare workers who have taken the same short course multiple times, or who have taken courses that do not relate to their duties. In many countries, a major source of healthcare-worker absenteeism is attendance at the courses! The proliferation of these courses has actually hampered healthcare-service delivery.

Compared to the more meaningful, in-depth work required to increase the numbers of healthcare workers, short-course training seems a quick, sure win. Creating new slots in existing schools involves improving the management, so that more students can be trained with the same resources; identifying additional clinical facilities where the students may do clinical practica; buying more materials (anatomical models, books, laboratory and medical equipment), and so on. Success takes a few years, not a few weeks.

Another wrinkle in the free-market approach is the existence of two types of demand for health workers. The free-market approach relies on supply and demand. But in healthcare there are two different types of demand. Most of us think of healthcare demand as the *need* for healthcare. In other words, sicker people have a greater demand, or need for healthcare. But the second type of demand is effective demand—the ability to pay for healthcare, in the US usually through health insurance. It is this second type of demand that drives healthcare-worker career and location choices and drives a mismatch between health needs and healthcare-worker supply.

Efforts by International and Bilateral Organizations

After a lull in attention to the global health workforce in the 1980s and 1990s, HIV/AIDS forced the issue back onto the international stage at the turn of the 21st century, as the disease devastated the populations of many developing countries. In Botswana, 23 percent of all adults were HIV positive; rates in some communities there approached 50 percent. India experienced the world's biggest epidemic: 2.4 million people there were infected with HIV/AIDS. To date, more than 40 million people around the globe have died from HIV/AIDS; 33 million are currently infected.

The global health community succeeded in placing over 5.2 million people cumulatively in developing countries on antiretroviral care. Such a rapid scale-up in complex medical treatment was unprecedented. To achieve this, incredible hurdles were overcome. Political opposition was addressed, and government leaders eventually acknowledged that HIV was present in their countries and that many of them, in fact, had lost loved ones to the disease. The social stigma began to fall away as discriminatory laws were removed, and opinion leaders—politicians, religious figures, pop stars—were photographed embracing people known to have HIV/AIDS. New and even better treatments were developed, and pharmaceutical companies were persuaded to sell their antiretroviral drugs to developing countries at cost and, despite active patents, to allow generic-drug manufacturers in those countries to manufacture the drugs.

Perhaps most remarkably, the effort to address HIV/AIDS resulted in a doubling of global health aid. Donor funding for HIV/AIDS in developing countries grew from $300 million in 1996[8] to $15.6 billion in 2008.[9] In just the four years between 2002 and 2006, donor funding for HIV/AIDS prevention, treatment, and care grew by 600 percent. In 2008, President Bush's President's Emergency Plan for AIDS Relief (PEPFAR) expressed commitments of $48 billion for the period 2009 to 2013, of which $39 billion has now been committed.[10]

But as HIV/AIDS became the most heavily funded disease in history, millions of dollars languished in bank accounts, because there weren't enough healthcare workers to deliver the services the money would pay for. With too few healthcare workers to diagnose and treat the disease, antiretroviral drugs expired on clinic shelves.[11] Every year, 2.7 million people are newly infected with HIV, while currently a total of only 4 million people in poor and middle-income countries have access to lifesaving antiretroviral therapy. Each year, the gap between the number of people with HIV/AIDS who need access to healthcare workers and those who have such access widens. The healthcare workforce remains the last unaddressed issue in the HIV/AIDS crisis.

Under these circumstances, it became clear that retraining primary healthcare workers to become HIV/AIDS workers was hugely insufficient. Not only was this short-course strategy not creating a single new healthcare worker; it was also causing a "rob Peter to pay Paul" situation, with healthcare workers being pulled from essential primary care to provide specialized AIDS care. This created an ethical dilemma: Adults with HIV/AIDS were being treated with complex drug regimens by highly trained teams of workers, while children died from lack of access to a healthcare worker who could treat their diarrhea.

And with more and more people infected each year, more and more healthcare workers were needed to care for them. In some countries, great numbers of healthcare workers were themselves dying from AIDS; others were becoming less productive because of their own HIV infection or from having to care for their extended-family members with HIV/AIDS.

In the late 1990s, under pressure from AIDS activists and members of developing countries affected by HIV/AIDS, the World Health Organization reconstituted its health-workforce unit. Recognizing that the majority of healthcare workers are women, thus giving the term "manpower planning" a negative connotation, the reconstituted entity was called the Health Workforce Unit. While the unit worked to fill the coordinating and standard-setting role that WHO had played, it was grossly underfunded compared to the need. Depending on the country and the healthcare system, healthcare-worker salaries can represent 60 to 85 percent of the healthcare budget—an enormous investment. So it might naturally follow that dealing with the healthcare workforce would represent a large portion of the WHO budget. But the Health Workforce Unit received just a tiny fraction of the overall budget. Charged with advising nearly 60 countries with healthcare-workforce shortages so acute they cannot even meet basic demands for primary care, the unit was itself severely understaffed, and its staffing has recently been cut again by more than two-thirds.

With donors setting aside only a small percentage of their funding to increase the global healthcare workforce, AIDS activists looked back at how they had achieved their unprecedented increase in funding and coordination. A key element in the success of the HIV/AIDS movement was a separate entity within the United Nations, UNAIDS, established in 1993 to coordinate global efforts to combat the disease. UNAIDS is an independent unit, outside WHO; its director, rather than reporting up through the WHO chain of command, reports to a board made up of representatives of UN agencies (including WHO) and UN member countries. With its increased flexibility and visibility, UNAIDS is able to give fundraising and action for HIV/AIDS a higher profile. WHO still maintains its own smaller internal HIV/AIDS unit.

Modeled somewhat after UNAIDS, a semi-independent unit, the Global Health Workforce Alliance, was created in 2006 to coordinate global efforts to address the healthcare-workforce crisis. As with UNAIDS, the executive director of the alliance reports directly to the WHO secretary general, as well as to an independent board whose members represent the most important current and potential health-workforce donors. These include the US government, the Bill and Melinda Gates Foundation, the government of Norway, the World Bank, and Physicians for Human Rights (representing nongovernmental organizations). The Global Health Workforce Alliance was tasked with a clear coordinating role: convening the community working on health workforce, advocating on their behalf, speeding the dissemination of information and the adoption of successful interventions, and preventing the duplication of work.

The alliance got off to a good start by signing up more than 100 member organizations, which gave it a powerful mandate to speak with one voice when advocating and fundraising. But its credibility was almost immediately compromised when, without consulting either its members or its board, the alliance announced a huge healthcare-worker education initiative. I remember receiving the e-mail announcement and immediately calling Dr. David Peters, the board member representing the World Bank at the time. He, too, had never heard of the initiative. Where would the millions of dollars for the initiative come from? we wondered. Who would receive the money, and how would it be spent? With fewer than five staff members, how would the alliance supervise such a large program?

Lacking answers to these questions, the alliance pulled the plug on the initiative. The sad part is that if the alliance had properly engaged its board and members, as well as global donors, in an effort to systematically expand the training of healthcare workers around the world, the initiative probably would have been well received. It could have received the funding and staffing it required to carry out such an ambitious and needed effort.

The alliance has never quite recovered from this mistake. It remains underfunded and understaffed. And it continues to focus on implementing healthcare-workforce reform, rather than on its intended purpose of coordinating advocacy, fundraising, and knowledge. Given its small budget, the alliance could have achieved far more by coordinating and maximizing the efforts of the other organizations in the field. Because it instead puts its limited resources toward implementing change, its contribution is too small to make much of a difference.

The alliance's flagship activity is assisting a set of eight "pathfinder" countries in implementing healthcare-workforce reform. But with its small budget, it has given only $100,000 to each country. Compared with the magnitude of the challenge—and the billions of dollars allocated to HIV/AIDS efforts—this is a pittance, especially given the size of some of the countries. The pathfinder country of Sudan (now split into two countries), for instance, has a population of 45 million people and is 2.5 million square kilometers, larger than the entire United States east of the Mississippi. The alliance has given Sudan, a country with some of the worst health statistics in the world, four cents per square mile, less than one cent per person, to help train, employ, and retain an adequate healthcare workforce.

Meanwhile, opportunities have been lost. In 2008, independently of one another, Japan and the United States—two of the world's largest global-health donors—announced massive commitments to training new healthcare workers in developing countries. Japan promised to train 100,000 healthcare workers; the United States, through PEPFAR, promised to train 140,000. Coordinating the work of the two countries and challenging other donors to make equal commitments would have been a perfect task for the alliance. The opportunity was not pursued, and so far, no similar donor commitments have been made.

Like WHO, the US government has not made the progress it would have liked in managing the global healthcare-worker shortage. Data is not publicly available on the progress made toward training those 140,000 healthcare workers. Even if this laudable goal is achieved, it is still a drop in the bucket: 3.5 percent of the 4 million global healthcare-worker deficit.

Too Much and Not Enough

Although highly laudable, sending developing countries pharmaceuticals, or offering short courses to the few healthcare workers the countries have managed to retain, can never make up for the past, ongoing, and predictably larger future loss of so many experienced workers. No matter how well trained and motivated, no one worker can do the work of three people. Drugs cannot be prescribed without physicians or nurse practitioners; they cannot be dispensed without pharmacists. This is especially true with HIV/AIDS medications. The United States has invested close to $39 billion[12] in the President's Emergency Plan for AIDS Relief, but the number one obstacle in AIDS treatment remains the lack of healthcare workers.

One of the few wealthy countries to address the consequences of its actions and more fully attempt to correct its massive healthcare-worker insourcing is the United Kingdom. In 2003 the United Kingdom and former colonies passed the Commonwealth Code of Practice for the International Recruitment of Health Workers, which prohibited national healthcare systems from directly recruiting from countries with healthcare-worker shortages. The code was not legally binding, however, and it had a major unforeseen loophole. The ban drove the recruitment companies to serve the United Kingdom's private health sector, where they could recruit for large numbers of private nursing homes—which are not part of Commonwealth national health systems—as well as for smaller numbers of private hospitals and clinics. In a parallel process, the United Kingdom made major investments in expanding the number of training slots for health professionals in the nation and now has dramatically reduced the number of health workers it recruits from developing countries for the National Health Service.

Most thinking and action by global healthcare-workforce experts has focused on the national level and on ministries of health—that is, after all, the level at which they are used to working. This has caused them to overlook other organizations that significantly affect the global flow of healthcare workers. These

Organizations with the Power to Address the Global Healthcare-Worker Shortage

About a dozen organizations possess the technical expertise, funding, and influence to affect the global healthcare-worker shortage, including the United Nations, government development agencies, private foundations, and nonprofit and faith-based organizations. Two multinational organizations relevant to the movement of healthcare workers from poor to wealthy countries are the International Labor Organization and the International Organization for Migration. The queen of the multinational institutions remains the World Health Organization, founded in 1946 as part of the United Nations family of institutions to be the global coordinating authority on health issues. The ministers of health from the 194 member nations oversee WHO through their annual World Health Assembly meetings, where they propose, debate, and pass resolutions on important health matters.

The World Bank, for which I coordinated the African Health Workforce Program for five years, is the largest nongovernment funder of healthcare in the world. The World Health Organization may have the convening and technical authority, but the World Bank has the money, as well as a unique economics- and market-based approach to healthcare. WHO and other health institutions take it for granted that healthcare is a worthwhile goal, but the World Bank funds only work that can be shown to improve a country's economy. It provides loans that must be repaid and grants that require countries to meet certain accounting and business standards.

Most wealthy countries are members and funders of the multinational organizations, but they have their own national funding agencies. The largest of these single-country funders ("bilaterals") is the United States Agency for International Development (USAID), which has an annual health budget of more than $5 billion.* Other significant funders include the British Department for International Development, the Japanese International Cooperation Agency, the German Organization for Technical Cooperation, and the Norwegian Agency for Development Cooperation.

The biggest of the foundations focusing on healthcare is the Gates Foundation, with a $30 billion endowment from Bill and Melinda Gates and Warren Buffett. It spends $3 billion a year, equivalent to what the US government spends through USAID. Other prominent foundations are the Rockefeller Foundation, the Aspen Institute, the John D. and Catherine T. MacArthur Foundation, and the Rotary Foundation.

Many nonprofit organizations also focus on health and the global health-worker shortage. Three of the most prominent are Save the Children, Merlin, and the nonprofit I work for, IntraHealth International. As nonprofits, these organizations raise money from foundations, the US government, individuals, and other funders to implement programs directly in developing countries.

* "USAID's Total Health Budget by Program Category and Bureau, FY 2009," USAID, accessed December 24, 2011, www.usaid.gov/our_work/global_health/home/Funding/fundingbydirectives.html.

organizations include regional- and global-cooperation entities such as the World Trade Organization, as well as non-health-related national ministries such as ministries of trade and commerce. A prime example of health workforce experts' collective blind spot is the European Commission's Bologna Process on Higher Education. Many healthcare experts saw no reason to pay much attention to an entity that oversees education until they learned that it may soon force European Community members to recognize the license of any healthcare worker with a degree from a school in an EC country—regardless of the language of instruction or the worker's proficiency in the language of the country in which he or she seeks to practice.

All this is done in the name of eliminating barriers to commerce. But there are concerns about this process throughout Europe. What the proposal means is that a Romanian or Bulgarian physician would be able to practice medicine in the United Kingdom or Germany without having to demonstrate any knowledge of that country's language, medical system, standards of care, or cultural preferences. Wealthier western European countries worry that they will be flooded with poorly trained doctors from poorer eastern European countries who will harm patients. And the poorer countries worry that they will lose a large percentage of their doctors to wealthier countries and be unable to provide basic health services. Caught off guard by this notion, health experts in EC countries are trying to insert language to guarantee some minimal set of competencies and to protect essential health services so that lives are not endangered.

A similar threat of opening the floodgates of health-worker migration exists under the World Trade Organization's General Agreement on Trade in Services (GATS). At present, the United States does not automatically recognize the degrees of healthcare workers from other countries. Instead, health workers trained overseas who wish to work in the United States must at minimum pass a licensing exam. The World Trade Organization views this as a barrier to free trade in services because it hinders Brazilian-trained physicians, say, from selling their services in the United States, the largest healthcare market in the world. If GATS continues on this course, the United States will be forced to allow any healthcare worker to practice here, regardless of his or her level of knowledge, English-language skills, or cultural competency.

In the face of the global healthcare-worker shortage, some countries and healthcare organizations, such as the International Council of Nurses, the East African Community, and the West African Science Campus, are advocating to set global or regional standards for healthcare-worker education. This would mean that a nursing or medical degree from any country would be recognized by other countries and that healthcare workers could practice in another country without having to verify their knowledge or skills.

The idea is that standardization would make it easier for surplus health workers to voluntarily leave their home countries and migrate to countries with health-worker shortages and thus even out health-worker densities. Past experience suggests, however, that rather than smoothing out health-worker densities, standardization will exaggerate them. Healthcare workers licensed to work in multiple countries will end up in the wealthier countries, where they can find the best wages and working environments, continuing professional development, and opportunities for their families. Standardization will exaggerate our existing problem, not solve it. If wealthy countries had never licensed foreign-trained physicians and nurses, those wealthy countries would have been forced to invest in their own people, and the developing world could have retained its healthcare workers.

Successful Efforts to Curb Insourcing

Some countries, including Thailand, Sri Lanka, the Philippines, and the United Kingdom, have examined their country's healthcare needs and invested in training the right number of the right type of healthcare workers to meet those needs. These cost-effective programs provide good models. In this country, a few—too few—states and schools have also found ways to increase the access to a healthcare education. It's a start.

When my husband and I honeymooned in Thailand in 1999, we had no idea we were in a country that had achieved a level of healthcare for its citizens comparable to that in the United States, with only a fraction of the wealth. Even though they live in a country with a gross domestic product of less than $4,000 per capita, Thais have an average life expectancy of 73 years. In the United States, with a per capita GDP of $46,000—more than 10 times higher—Americans have an average life expectancy of 78 years, just five years more.

From the isolated hill tribes in the north to the small fishing villages in the south, Thais have excellent access to physicians. Thailand has long had fine medical-training programs and good numbers of students who want to become physicians. Indeed, it used to be an excellent source of physicians for the US market. In the 1960s, more than one-third of new medical school graduates left Thailand, mainly to practice in the United States.[1] This was a considerable loss to the country. Not only did the Thais lose a vast number of graduating physicians; they also lost a significant financial investment: In Thailand, medical students pay only 5 percent of the real cost of their training. The government subsidizes the rest, and there was no way to recoup this investment when the physicians migrated.

In the past, Thai city dwellers had 21 times the number of physicians per capita than those who lived in poor and rural areas. Many rural and poor communities had no doctor at all. In the 1970s, however, the government realized that the health of its citizens plays a significant role in a nation's economic growth and political stability—that access to healthcare workers is important not just to individuals and communities but to the country as a whole. Noting the global evidence that students from rural backgrounds are more likely to practice in their home communities, the government started a series of reforms to decrease the number of doctors who emigrated and increase the number of physicians working in underserved areas.

The new policies and programs worked so well that the number of medical students from rural backgrounds increased quickly and dramatically, from less than 6 percent of all medical school graduates in 1974 to more than 45 percent in 1983, without compromising the quality of the graduates. The total number of physicians in Thailand doubled.[2] Such a rapid increase is nothing new. As mentioned earlier, the United States doubled its production of physicians during World War II. So many physicians had been deployed to the war effort that more were needed to care for people at home, as well as to save lives on the front lines. Like the factories running day and night, the medical schools increased their output by making classes bigger and eliminating the months-long summer breaks.

Much of Thailand's increase in physicians came through new medical schools, opened mainly in underserved areas. Students living in those areas could pursue their studies close to their families and maintain ties with their communities, which increased their likelihood of returning to those communities to practice. And the students who came from elsewhere developed ties and experience in the community; as the evidence shows, students who train in underserved communities are more likely to practice in them.[3]

The Thais also worked to increase the career and economic rewards of being a rural physician. They created a series of annual awards for the best rural doctors, to provide recognition for their work, and offered retention incentives—that is, bonuses—to physicians working in rural areas. Perhaps more important, they developed greater career-advancement opportunities in rural areas. To give one example, directors of rural hospitals are the career equivalent of a deputy director general in the central Ministry of Health, a senior and extremely prestigious position.

In less than 10 years, the combination of all these interventions and incentives decreased the imbalance in numbers of urban and rural physicians, from 21 to just 8.6 times more physicians per capita in urban areas. This led to an improvement in health status. The overall infant-mortality rate in Thailand, for instance, dropped from 55 deaths per 1,000 live births to 40 deaths per 1,000 live births.

New Approaches in the Philippines and Sri Lanka

What has happened in healthcare-worker education in the Philippines is nothing short of revolutionary. With the country's long history of high unemployment, the government decided to promote access to higher education and to lower barriers to the opening of private colleges. Since 1990, the Philippines has more than doubled its nurse-training capacity at almost no cost to the government—mainly through the opening of private and faith-based colleges.

These private nursing colleges in the Philippines rely on students paying off their student loans once they begin working. This strategy means the schools have to perform: If their graduates cannot pass their licensing exams or get jobs, they can't pay back the money they owe. Moreover, students will stop seeking out a school with a poor reputation, and it might have to close. In the United States, however, public colleges and universities that do not deliver on their obligations, like financial institutions that are "too big to fail," tend to receive *more* money, which is like investing in a falling stock. In the Philippines, the private nursing schools must compete on price, so they have to focus on the cost-effectiveness of each aspect of their programs. The true miracle of that country's increased production of nurses is that tuition at the private nursing schools is affordable for most Filipino families.

One of the most incredible successes in providing adequate numbers of healthcare workers, and distributing them where they are most needed, is Sri Lanka. In just three years, between 1947 and 1950, Sri Lanka (then Ceylon) was able to cut its maternal-mortality rate in half and to make significant improvement in its infant-mortality rates. The country has maintained that success. In 2008, the maternal-mortality rate was 39 deaths per 100,000 live births, compared with 540 deaths per 100,000 births in India. (The United States has 17 maternal deaths per 100,000 live births.) This occurred despite a prolonged and active civil war and while Sri Lanka spent less on healthcare ($29 per person) than most other countries do. The United States spends an annual average of $4,271 per person on healthcare. That's almost as much as Sri Lanka's entire GDP per capita, which is $4,500 per year.

The key to increasing access to healthcare workers came mainly through creating a new type of worker: the family-health worker, who visits every woman during her pregnancy, as well as for a period of time after the child's birth. Sri Lanka's success demonstrates that all countries can become less reliant on expensive, high-level healthcare workers, domestic or imported, by increasing the use of frontline healthcare workers, who live and work near those most in need.

How the United Kingdom Reduced Its Dependence on Foreign Healthcare Workers

An organization whose size is superseded by only the Chinese army and the Indian Rail System, Britain's National Health Service is the world's largest single employer of healthcare workers. Less than a decade ago, that system was heavily dependent on foreign medical school graduates, just as in the United States. This lack of investment in its own youth was particularly surprising because about one-third of the households in the United Kingdom depend on the government for 50 percent of their income.

As we have seen in earlier chapters, the United Kingdom's colonial links facilitated the emigration of healthcare professionals from those countries. Before 2008, almost half of the physicians in the National Health Service were foreign trained—and, worse, the majority were from WHO health-workforce-crisis countries, such as India, Malawi, Nigeria, and Zambia. As the governments of these countries began to realize they were unable to improve the health of their peoples because they were losing their most qualified healthcare workers, they began to pressure the United Kingdom to stop importing so many workers.

Of course, it was easier to convey their dissatisfaction to the United Kingdom than it has been to do so with the United States. As part of the British Commonwealth (the United Kingdom and 53 of its former colonies, not including the United States), the countries losing their healthcare workers to Britain could directly address the issue. In addition, the United Kingdom is a much smaller aid donor.

By 1998, the United Kingdom was bringing in so many foreign-trained physicians that British-trained physicians were having trouble finding residency positions and jobs. Faced with pressure at home as well as from abroad, the National Health Service began investing in training more physicians domestically. In just 10 years, the number of medical school slots doubled.[4] Once the number of graduates doubled, the United Kingdom stopped importing foreign-trained physicians almost entirely.

A Few Encouraging Examples in the United States: Rural Programs

In this country, most healthcare workers spend the majority of their training in hospital wards—even though less than 5 percent of patients can be found there—and most teaching hospitals are in metropolitan areas. No wonder there is a mismatch between this country's healthcare needs and the skills of the healthcare workers we train. The United States could certainly learn some lessons from Thailand, Sri Lanka, and the Philippines.

But you can find programs that align healthcare-worker training with local health needs in this country, too. Pennsylvania has been at the forefront of such efforts, particularly in underserved rural communities. Of all 50 states, Pennsylvania has the third-largest number of rural residents. One-half of all the physicians practicing in that state work in just three counties; the other half cover the remaining 64 counties, where three-quarters of the population lives. In addition to this physician-to-population imbalance, the average age, and thus the average healthcare needs, are far higher in the rural counties.

As bad as these statistics sound, things would be much worse if not for the Physician Shortage Area Program (PSAP). In 1974, the Pennsylvania state government and Jefferson Medical College, at Thomas Jefferson University, in Philadelphia, created this program to train medical students for careers as family physicians in the state's underserved rural areas. Every element of the program is designed to produce the type of healthcare worker who can meet the health needs of rural communities.

PSAP runs parallel with Jefferson's standard medical school program. The two sets of students take the same scientific courses, but their expectations, clinical experience, and mentors are quite different. This alignment of training and eventual service begins with admissions: The PSAP program gives preference to students from rural areas who express a desire to work in rural communities and have a demonstrated history of serving these communities. Although PSAP participants are not legally bound to work in rural areas on graduation, they are given the distinct sense that they are pledging to serve these communities—that if they go on to pursue a career in a metropolitan area or in specialty care, their credibility will be compromised.

The program pairs each PSAP student with a mentor practicing family medicine in rural Pennsylvania. The mentors help these students understand the unique rewards associated with taking care of the health needs of families and entire communities, from delivering a newborn to providing palliative care to the child's great-grandmother. In their third and fourth years of medical school, during their clinical rotations, PSAP students spend less time in hospitals and intensive-care units in favor of more time in primary-care clinics and on home visits.

This eliminates one barrier to expanding the number of medical school students. Many healthcare-professional schools claim they cannot accept more students each year because they do not have access to enough sites for clinical rotations. Expanding the rotation experience beyond the hospital and into community-based clinics, which is where most patients are, can certainly increase student capacity. And, recognizing that every program looking for a specific type of person needs a good pipeline, PSAP has established relationships with several rural colleges in the state so that the program can interest high-achieving rural students in considering careers in rural medicine. With these connections and its efforts in raising the profile and image of rural physicians, PSAP does not have to compromise when it admits students.

This intelligent plan and program has paid off. A 2008 study found that even though they represent just 1 percent of the graduates from Pennsylvania's seven medical schools, PSAP graduates account for 21 percent of the family physicians practicing in rural Pennsylvania.[5] The program has been so successful that the neighboring state of Delaware has provided funding for PSAP to recruit and train young people from that state's rural communities.

Pennsylvania has been innovative in other ways, too. For example, in response to recent spikes in general unemployment, as well as to the high vacancy rates in the nursing field, the state government teamed up with private-sector organizations to increase funding for nursing schools—particularly for hiring more faculty and increasing student capacity. Most of the private-sector money came from hospitals, which are finally starting to recognize that the lack of nurses costs them money in recruiting fees and lost business. Other private funding came from non-healthcare-related businesses that felt they were having trouble attracting employees because of the shortage of available healthcare in their communities.

Meeting the Health Needs of Minority Communities

The health disparities between minority communities, particularly African American and Latino communities, and the general population are great. To cite just one example, a 2004 study found that African American infants are twice as likely to die in the first year of life as the average American infant.[6] African American women are more than four times more likely to die of childbirth-related complications than white women are; the average life span of African Americans is almost five years shorter than that of whites.[7] One way to begin decreasing these disparities is to train more minority Americans to serve in the healthcare field.

Many studies have shown that, just as with rural communities, minority healthcare workers are more likely to live and work in their own communities. According to the Association of American Medical Colleges, African American physicians are five times more likely to serve African American communities than physicians of other races are. They serve higher proportions of uninsured and underinsured patients; nearly half their patients are uninsured or on Medicaid, which pays far lower rates than private health insurance. African American, Latino, and Native American physicians are also more likely to conduct research addressing the health challenges of minority communities.[8]

Traditionally, most minority healthcare workers have been

trained in African American colleges and universities. But, just as Jefferson Medical College developed a special program to train physicians for rural areas, a few US medical schools have created programs to identify high-achieving minority students. One such school is the University of Tennessee, in Knoxville. Once ranked very low in terms of minority admissions — in the bottom 25 percent of medical schools — it is now in the top 25 percent, thanks to the Tennessee Institutes for Pre-Professionals (TIP), a program created by the university to identify and support underrepresented minority students.

The TIP program provides opportunities for minority students interested in careers in medicine, pharmacy, and dentistry to be paired with a mentor in their field of interest and gain some exposure to what it's like to work in that field. TIP helps interested students prepare for the medical, pharmacy, or dental school admissions tests and prepares them for the types of courses they will encounter.

Similar programs — such as one at the University of California that works with minority students between college graduation and the time they apply for medical school — have been successful in expanding the enrollment of young minority women and men in medical schools. Some programs start with children as young as middle school; other programs guarantee medical school admission to high school and college undergraduates who meet their requirements, such as maintaining a certain grade-point average and participating in educational summer programs. The city of Camden, New Jersey, has the Dr. Charles Brimm Medical Arts High School, which encourages high-achieving students from minority and low-income households to enter the health professions.

Despite the success of programs like TIP, most minority healthcare workers, including Latinos, continue to be trained in large part at the 103 Historically Black Colleges and Universities, such as Howard University, in Washington, DC; Spelman College, in Atlanta; and Xavier University of Louisiana, in New Orleans. Similarly, Hispanic-Serving Institutions (HSIs) represent just 6 percent of all postsecondary schools yet enroll roughly half of all Latino students. Tribal Colleges and Universities educate the majority of Native Americans in health careers. For rural communities there are the Area Health Education Centers (AHECs) and Rural Medicine programs. If we are going to reduce healthcare disparities by training more healthcare workers from minority and rural communities, we also need to give more support to these institutions to enable them to expand their programs.

Reducing the Cost of Training

If we could bring down the cost of educating healthcare workers, we could train more workers. The total cost of training healthcare workers has been increasing more rapidly than inflation. That is unsustainable, and there is little evidence that the cost-effectiveness of care is improved by constantly adding more and more expensive requirements to practice.

An excellent example of cost reduction is the nurse-training program at Cedar Crest College, in Allentown, Pennsylvania. Taking nurse-training programs out of hospitals and putting them into colleges and universities was the single greatest reason for the jump in training costs for nurses. Unlike the students in medical and most other health-professional schools, students in typical nursing programs must take a professor with them when they do their clinical rotations. One professor must accompany every four students, from schools that might have a hundred students in a single class. Obviously, this practice dramatically increases the number of nursing professors required.

And nursing professors need a master's degree, which is beyond the profession's basic requirements. Rather than expanding the profession, this practice creates an additional bottleneck. Not allowing senior nurses to supervise nursing students is a major reason for the rise in the cost of a nursing education. It is the main and unrecognized cause of the nursing-faculty shortage.

In an effort to make nursing education more affordable for students and for the college, Cedar Crest formed relationships with neighboring hospitals in which nursing students might gain exposure to the work. Staff nurses were trained to become "clinical associates" and supervise the nursing students on their clinical practica and provide training in essential, practical skills, such as responding to emergencies, assessing patients, administering medicine, and communicating with the rest of the health-care team.

Overseen by the clinical associates, nursing students are allowed to work in the wards at no additional cost to the school. With more nursing hands, the hospitals can provide better quality of care and use the program as a recruiting tool. The school benefits because it can increase its student capacity at minimal cost. Most research on the subject has shown that health-care students are more likely to work in an institution in which they did some of their training. The community benefits because more of its young people can enter an expanding field, and more nurses are available to care for the community.

Problems regarding the number and distribution of health-care workers are not insurmountable. A common thread running through the programs I have described is the political will to make a change. All it takes is for all the parties involved to work together to realize that goal.

The Way Forward

The US healthcare-worker shortage will not be solved with initiatives focused on foreign healthcare workers. Only by fixing its own system will the United States be able to wean itself off its reliance on insourced foreign health workers. It will not be easy, but it can be done. Achieving workforce self-sufficiency in America's largest economic sector will require the coordinated efforts of healthcare institutions, universities, citizen groups, and federal, state, and local governments.

As a pediatrician serving some of the poorest communities in the United States and as a healthcare policy expert at the global level, I have examined many potential solutions to the healthcare-worker crisis. I have had the benefit of experiencing firsthand hundreds of different proposed and implemented solutions, in all types of settings—from rich to poor, urban to rural, democratic to autocratic—in systems ranging from centralized national to market based. I've seen approaches as different as the new Ethiopian strategy of flooding the market for healthcare workers, in the hope that sufficient numbers will stay in country, and the Thai requirement of a period of national service in primary care in underserved areas. As I have traveled the world helping countries with their healthcare-worker shortages, my mind has constantly traveled back to my own—to this country's pivotal role in the global maldistribution and shortage of healthcare workers, and to what we can do to provide every American with a decent level of healthcare.

It is not enough for a solution to be technically correct; it must also be acceptable from the political, economic, and cultural point of view. There is no shortage of technically feasible policy proposals gathering dust in file cabinets because they were not affordable or could not get the backing of healthcare workers, legislators, or the general public. Here is what I think the United States should do to address its healthcare-worker maldistribution and shortage—and, in the process, to lead the world by example.

Train More Healthcare Workers

Without a doubt, the most important thing the United States can do is to invest in its own citizens and train more healthcare workers. Globally only 1.8 percent of all healthcare expenditures are invested in health-worker education. The United States spends only one-third of that, 0.5 percent of healthcare expenditures, on health-worker education.[1] That is a surprisingly small investment in the education of the people who make the decisions in our nation's largest and fastest-growing economic sector. What is needed now is similar to the World War II increase in production of health workers. For at least the next few decades, our production of nurses, nurse practitioners, pharmacists, behavior-change workers, and almost all other healthcare professionals will have to increase by at least 50 percent more than our current production. In general, the production of doctors will need to increase by at least 25 percent, and we'll need to double the number of primary-care doctors. As in any emergency situation, the rules will need to change, and we'll need to train more health workers better, faster, and more cost-efficiently.

Later on, I will address how we will finance this massive investment in our own people.

We need not fear training too many healthcare workers. If it appears that we have overcompensated and are training too many workers in a particular field, it is relatively easy to reduce the numbers of students entering the training programs. If the newly trained workers cannot find clinical positions, many or most should be able to find work in administrative, policy, or leadership positions within the healthcare sector.

Finding the sites to train more healthcare workers is far easier than it may seem. Most classrooms and labs in health-science schools are empty more often than they are full. At the Johns Hopkins University School of Medicine, students are in class only during the morning hours; the school could easily double its output of physicians by running classes in the afternoon, too. The Johns Hopkins University School of Nursing has already done this, doubling the number of graduates each year and giving a second group of students the reverse classroom-clinic schedule as the original cohort.

The United States has no shortage of medical school professors. Doctors clamor for an opportunity to combine patient care with teaching at academic hospitals, even though academic medical salaries are lower than those in nonacademic settings. Finding professors to teach all the new nursing students should not be a problem if we give nursing professors the flexibility enjoyed by most med school professors, who spend a fraction of their time teaching. They could augment their salaries through clinical and management work. As for their salaries, if we increased them to something near what clinical work pays, we would rapidly have enough nursing professors. Dropping the requirement for nursing professors to have degrees two levels above the qualifying degree of nursing and making use of expert nurse clinicians in the community will also dramatically expand the numbers of nurses who can teach nursing students.

How we go about dramatically expanding our production of healthcare workers will make all the difference in the world. Every health-professional school should create an employer advisory board that includes representatives from the institutions, such as clinics, hospitals, and nursing homes that will eventually employ its graduates. As schools ramp up their programs, this employer advisory board will ensure they are recruiting and training the types of workers that employers most want to hire. Are local employers looking to hire super-subspecialty MD/PhDs to do research in academic hospitals? Or are they looking for primary-care doctors, nurse practitioners, and physician assistants, especially to work in underserved communities?

The next four proposals concern the types of students that schools should recruit and the types of healthcare workers the schools should produce.

Train More Primary-Care Workers

While the United States has a shortage of all healthcare workers, including specialists, the lack of primary-care providers has the most dire consequences for our health. The shortage will become even more acute as health-insurance coverage increases and as the country ages. We must make sure that the proportion of generalists to specialists becomes larger.

Most research indicates that at least 50 percent of all healthcare workers in the country should be generalists. Since generalists can be trained and employed more quickly—and thus less expensively—than specialists, this will reduce the per capita cost of healthcare. This recommendation shouldn't be hard to institute. Schools will be guided by employment advisory boards on the number of generalists to train and the ratio of generalists to specialists. If universities listen to what employers are looking for, they will train more primary-care workers. Local, state, and federal governments can use incentives or set goals for the number of generalists trained by schools receiving their funding. Federal and state funding for healthcare-worker education should be aligned with our healthcare priorities and go to primary-care cadres, such as nurse practitioners and physician assistants, as well as to medical schools and residencies that graduate a large number of physicians who go into primary care.

We also need to improve on efforts to adjust the reimbursement rates that insurers pay for primary-care services versus specialty services. Rather than adding new money, we can begin to balance out the payment differentials between the two. Insurers should also balance the pay differentials they pay for services in metropolitan versus rural areas. Under current reimbursement rates, an OB/GYN physician would be paid more to deliver a baby in Miami than in rural Montana. This practice was initially meant to account for different costs of living, but it has transformed into a powerful disincentive to practice in rural areas.

Train More Midlevel Providers

The United States has a physician-heavy healthcare system. Yet, in both primary and specialty care, the vast majority of patients can be cared for by midlevel providers: physician assistants, nurse practitioners, nurse midwives, and advanced-practice nurses. As a primary-care pediatrician, I realized early on that less than 10 percent of my patients need my 10-plus years of postsecondary training and full physician skills. Multiple studies have shown that for the majority of patients, nurse practitioners and physician assistants can provide high-quality care at a lower cost.[2] The healthcare team should reflect this reality.

The community clinic in which I practice has five pediatricians and two nurse practitioners. Given that most patient visits are for well-child checkups, simple colds, and common childhood ailments, this physician-based team doesn't make sense; it is neither cost effective nor a good division of labor. A more rational staffing would be one pediatrician and eight nurse practitioners. The physician would care for patients whose diagnoses and treatments are complicated or uncommon and provide technical supervision for the nurse practitioners. Even with the additional two people on staff, the salary costs would be roughly the same. But the clinic could see a greater number of patients in our underserved community.

Strategic use of midlevel providers delivers many benefits. Perhaps most important, these providers, too, can be trained in a fraction of the time it takes to train a physician. The most basic primary-care physician has 11 years of higher education. Physician assistants can be trained in less than two years. Nurse practitioners can be trained in less than five years. To become an advanced-practice nurse, an RN needs to study for only an additional two years. The shorter training time is reflected in the reduced cost of training. It costs $400,000 to train a nurse practitioner, as opposed to the total cost of around $1 million to train a physician. And, correspondingly, salaries for midlevel providers are lower. Nurse practitioners and physician assistants make 60 to 70 percent of what most physicians earn.

In addition, midlevel healthcare providers are more likely than high-level providers to work in underserved communities, where the clinics and hospitals offer wages more in line with midlevel providers' salaries than with those for physicians. Although midlevel providers can specialize, most do not; and when they do, they provide specialty care at a lower cost.

Americans will not have to compromise on healthcare quality as coverage expands. Studies show that for annual physicals and the management of common illnesses, midlevel providers offer care that is equal or superior to that provided by physicians. And patient satisfaction levels are often higher: Since their salaries are lower, midlevel providers can spend more time with each patient. This frees both primary-care physicians and specialist physicians to focus on the more complicated patients and tasks in their work.

Train and Employ More Behavior-Change Healthcare Workers

My husband is among the 65 percent of American adults who are overweight. Like many of them, he has high blood pressure associated with his weight. Our current healthcare-workforce model provides him with an internist and a cardiologist, whom he sees twice a year. He has seen them for the past five years, and guess what? He is still overweight, and he still has high blood pressure. If we had a healthcare-workforce model that supported prevention in addition to treatment, he would be healthier and spend less money on healthcare.

Our health depends greatly on our behavior: what we eat and drink, how much we exercise, how we handle stress, whether or not we smoke or use illegal drugs, how consistently we take our prescribed medications. Physicians normally do not have time to address these issues with their patients, nor is it in their skill set. By themselves, only one in five adults reports being successful in a major health-related behavior change, such as quitting smoking or eating better, according to the American Psychological Association. This type of change is much more easily made with ongoing professional support.[3] But our healthcare system is not structured to provide this support.

There is a solution. In Europe, around the world, and even in parts of the United States, frontline behavior-change workers have had considerable success. Because these workers do not need college degrees (their training usually takes a year or less) but can be extremely helpful, they are more cost effective than physicians and nurses in changing behavior. Behavior-change workers can come to clients' homes to help them develop diet and exercise plans, show them how to cook, and remind them to take their medicine. They can check in frequently by phone to offer encouragement and help their clients overcome obstacles, such as the holiday-eating season. My husband would be greatly helped in his weight-loss efforts if a community healthcare worker called him a few times a week to see how his dieting and exercise regimen was going.

Behavior-change workers who focus on very common diagnoses with potentially high cost complications—diabetes, for instance, or high-risk newborns and their mothers—can master their subject in just a few months. Their training is practical rather than theoretical. A frontline healthcare worker does not need to understand the chemical structure of insulin to help a diabetic make better food choices and understand how to calculate her insulin doses. It would be far too expensive for a doctor or advanced-practice nurse to regularly take a couple of hours to review with a diabetic how to measure her blood-sugar level, determine how much insulin to take, and administer the dose. And frontline healthcare workers do more than help people manage their illnesses and live healthier lives. Because they have more frequent contact with patients, they can help identify problems more quickly, ensuring that the patient receives the care of a higher-level healthcare worker before the problem becomes more serious and more costly to address.

Doctors mainly diagnose and treat disease; frontline healthcare workers prevent disease and injury from occurring or from getting worse. A nurse educator or community healthcare worker who helps a diabetic keep his or her sugar under control and prevents a single hospitalization saves the healthcare system more than the cost of his or her annual salary: A single hospital stay can cost tens of thousands of dollars. Training more of these workers will yield a strong return on investment, in both lower healthcare costs and improved health around the country.

With their emphasis on prevention rather than curative care, behavior-change workers are essential to the healthcare system. Since they can be trained relatively quickly, the supply of these workers can be much more flexible, adjusted quickly in response to changing needs. As these workers become more common, we should see fewer physician and nurse visits. That means we will need to train and employ fewer physicians and nurses, which will lead to even greater cost savings.

The major barrier to the widespread use of behavior-change workers is that many insurance companies do not reimburse for their services. Medicare and Medicaid can lead the way in reimbursing for such services—and provide even more evidence that the use of behavior-change workers lowers overall healthcare costs.

Align Student Recruitment and Training with Healthcare Needs

We need to align our healthcare workforce with our national needs. A look at who is being recruited and admitted into US medical and nursing schools gives the impression that the purpose of the healthcare-education system is to train white people to do medical research in metropolitan academic centers. Whites make up 64 percent of the population. Even though they are the healthiest large segment of the population, almost three-quarters (74 percent) of the country's physicians are white. While 20 percent of the population lives in rural areas, less than 10 percent of medical students are from rural backgrounds. Latinos and African Americans make up 16 percent and 12 percent, respectively, of the US population, but only 4 percent and 5 percent of the total number of doctors.[4] No wonder African American, Latino, Native American, and rural communities have the least access to healthcare workers and also have the highest disease burdens.

We must make recruitment and admissions evidence-based and adjust our recruitment and admissions criteria to address the unserved needs of so many people. As we have already seen, countless studies have shown that nurses and doctors who grow up in rural communities are more likely to work in rural communities. That is even without bonding, or what I prefer to call return service, when, in exchange for financial aid, students agree to serve a certain period of time in an area where they are most needed. Such evidence must be taken into account when designing admissions criteria for schools that receive local, state, or federal funding.[5]

At present, grades and test scores reign supreme in medical school and nursing school admissions. But having genius doctors in ivory towers hundreds of miles away does underserved communities little good. What these communities need are local healthcare workers. If the United States is ever going to rise from *last position* in the health rankings of wealthy countries, we must have competent healthcare workers in every community. A background in an underserved community, a stated desire to serve that community, and evidence of having served it in other ways should be important factors in admission to any health-sciences school. Some may claim that this would lower the bar for admissions. But a system that produces workers who refuse to serve those most in need is a broken system.

Others might argue that telemedicine—using electronic communications and information technologies for clinical care—will eliminate the need to have healthcare workers in every community. A systematic review, however, found that telemedicine interventions are not more cost effective than the face-to-face provision of healthcare.[6] With improvements in remote cameras and listening devices, some follow-up primary-care visits could be done remotely. Telemedicine can work well with some specialties, such as radiology and dermatology. But for most other types of healthcare, you really need to have the patient in front of you to conduct a thorough examination and make a proper diagnosis.

Demographic and background characteristics are not the only factors affecting where health workers choose to practice. A large body of data shows that school location and exposure to underserved areas also affect this decision. Because people are more likely to live and work in their home communities, healthcare-training institutions should give preference to local applicants.[7]

But we must give all healthcare students the opportunity to work with underserved communities. Since most medical and nursing schools are located in major metropolitan areas, few students ever care for rural patients. As the number of health-sciences schools expands, we should make sure that many of them are located in areas with severe healthcare-worker shortages. The Bureau of Primary Health Care, in the US Department of Health and Human Services, already designates areas in which there are health-professional shortages.[8] So it will be easy to identify the most underserved communities and start opening health-professional schools there.

Reduce the Cost of Healthcare-Worker Education

The cost of education is the number one reason the United States does not train an adequate number of healthcare workers. The cost for an education in any profession of healthcare is increasing faster than inflation and wages, so continuing to train even the same number of students each year will become unsustainable. Much of the 2009 conversation on healthcare reform revolved around the concept of "bending the cost curve," meaning that we need to slow the rate of increase in the cost of healthcare compared with economic growth and inflation. Otherwise, the costs will soon outstrip our ability to pay. In the same way, we need to bend the cost curve for training healthcare workers. At the very least, we should prevent the cost of healthcare-worker education from rising any faster.

As the first step in keeping education costs under control, we need to set a new standard for regulating healthcare-training programs. Any mandatory changes to training programs should meet two important requirements: significant improvement in patient health and cost-effectiveness. Before the regulatory board of any healthcare profession can add a requirement—requiring a doctorate to practice, for instance—the board should demonstrate that the change will have an impact on quality of care sufficiently large to warrant the increase in the cost of training.

We can also reduce the cost of health-worker training by putting American creativity and business acumen to use. Texas governor Rick Perry has challenged the University of Texas system to create a $10,000 bachelor's degree. We should rise to this challenge with a $10,000 Registered Nursing degree, a $50,000 pharmacy degree, and a $75,000 medical degree. We will need to go further than the tuition cost; we will need to push down the overall real cost of the education. This can be accomplished through more efficient management of school resources and eliminating unnecessary content in curricula. Curricula for training healthcare professionals should be reexamined. Any classes or labs unnecessary for a clinical practice should be reduced or removed. That would shorten the time needed for training and make getting that education more affordable. Almost everyone I spoke to about the high cost of health-worker education cited the linkage with research as a major cost driver. The extra cost of researchers' salaries, lab space, and equipment is not covered by the grants they bring in. Yet less than 10 percent of our health workers engage in research as their primary occupation. Why are we pricing ourselves out of the clinicians we need by churning out researchers who end up being bored in clinical work? Eighty percent of all healthcare costs flow from the pen of a physician. Why are we training them to prefer to use the most expensive technologies possible? Not to mention the irony that since our research orientation means we can't afford to train enough health workers, we fill these empty posts with graduates from foreign schools that are of even lower quality and do less research than the most basic clinical-oriented school in the United States. There's no logic in that.

The United States is currently the global leader in the lucrative biomedical industry, and we should continue to seek to dominate this growing field. As we continue to shift from a heavy manufacturing economy to a high-tech economy, the children of steel-mill workers will find jobs helping to produce new treatments for currently untreatable cancers, brain disorders, and genetic diseases. But these workers can be taught in special research-oriented schools, not in every single health-professional school in the country.

There currently are medical schools that have more of a clinical and primary-care focus. Most of these are osteopathic medical schools, which grant a Doctor of Osteopathy (DO) degree rather than a Medical Doctorate (MD). There is no difference in the licensing or regulation between DOs and MDs. They take the same licensing exams and board exams. The difference is that it costs 25 percent less to train DOs, and they are more likely to enter primary care and serve rural communities and underserved populations. More of what we need, with a smaller price tag!

Most countries have six-year med school programs, which combine undergraduate and medical school. This model is not unknown in the United States, where there are almost 30 six-year medical school programs.[9] There should be far more. These programs provide more efficient training than the traditional eight-year programs and save an estimated $100,000 per student.[10]

An obvious way to reduce the cost of healthcare-worker education is to eliminate credential creep. For decades, audiologists, physical therapists, and nurse practitioners with master's degrees have provided high-quality care. They don't need to have doctorates. In order to increase the practice requirements for a profession, that profession should be able to demonstrate (1) that there currently are adequate numbers of that profession, (2) that they are well distributed throughout the country, (3) that the added expense of training and increased wages will be more than paid for in improved health outcomes for patients, and (4) that the added barrier to practice will not affect access to the care provided by that profession.

No matter how we increase the amount of money going into health-worker education, we need to use existing evidence to ensure that it goes toward creating the right kind of *additional* schools and slots that will meet America's health needs and is not just poured into the existing overpriced slots.

Overhaul the Way Healthcare-Worker Training Is Funded

The United States spends $15.6 billion per year on health-worker education. That's less than is spent on prescription drugs ($216 billion) or NIH research ($29.5 billion). Healthcare-worker education is funded through federal, state, and local educational subsidies to schools, private giving (such as donations to schools from alumni and others), federal government tuition loans, and direct tuition payments made by students and their families. If, over the next few years, we are going to increase healthcare-worker training by 50 percent or more, additional sources of funding must be found.

The United States is the only developed country that expects its young people to pay for significant portions of their education. As medical school tuition has increased, fewer students, especially those from poorer families, can afford to attend, at least not without taking out even larger loans. Since students have to worry about paying back all that money, increasing medical school debt burdens makes going into specialty care more enticing, even necessary. Enlarging the proportion of healthcare-training costs paid by the student is not the answer. The federal, state, and local governments need to put more money into healthcare-worker education, especially into the education of primary-care and midlevel providers.

This does not have to be new money. Every year the federal government gives over $100 billion in educational loans, including some to students studying for degrees with over 15 percent unemployment. We could align federal funding with national priorities and allocate a large percentage of this funding for health-professional programs. The money could come out of programs that have lower employment rates for their graduates.

Another existing funding stream that could be converted into funding to train additional health workers is unemployment insurance and jobs training money. Every year the United States spends more than $60 billion on unemployment benefits and $18 billion on federal jobs programs. Given that the health sector is the largest sector with open jobs and the sector predicted to experience the most job growth in the future, it makes sense to align our spending with job availability and needs. Since there are almost 100 different professions within the healthcare industry, there is a profession for every personality and intellectual ability. Since most healthcare-professional training takes less than four years, even older workers can have a meaningful career that makes the educational investment worthwhile.

Midcareer and older workers make very good candidates for scaling up health-worker training in the United States. I have had personal experience with three people who entered the health field in midcareer and made significant contributions. My high school chemistry teacher, Ms. Kathy Findley, after launching hundreds of students into health careers, decided to launch her own healthcare career. After spending over a decade teaching, she pursued a degree in pharmacy. Ms. Findley worked in the medical intensive care unit of a veteran's hospital for 10 years and now works for a pharmacology company. One of my fellow residents at Children's National Medical Center, Dr. Eric Rosenthal, had worked for 14 years in local and federal politics, serving as a congressional staffer and political director for the Human Rights Campaign Fund. Then he had an experience that changed his life. During the early years of the US AIDS epidemic, he and his partner adopted a boy with HIV. Interacting with the medical system in order to get the best care for his son compelled Eric to pursue a career in medicine. At an age when most physicians are already well established in their careers, Eric went to medical school and became a pediatrician. He currently sees patients in the Emergency Department at Children's National Medical Center and is a leading voice in the Washington, DC, pediatric community, championing healthcare for foster children and abused children. My children's own pediatrician, Dr. Barbara Stevens, was a computer programmer in her first career. After meeting her husband, a health economist, she became immersed in the world of healthcare. Realizing that healthcare was her true calling, she switched from high-tech to high-touch and now has her own growing practice.

And the private sector should contribute, too. Since a large driver of the cost of health-worker education is its links with biomedical research, why not ask the very pharmaceutical, biotech, and medical device companies that benefit to pay for the human capital that ensures their industry's success? Or why not ask health-sector employers to pay a certain amount into a healthcare-worker education fund whenever they hire a healthcare worker, whether a new grad or a seasoned professional? The amount would be proportional to the cost of educating the worker and would represent the true cost of the inputs to their industry: A hospital or clinic might pay $15,000 if it hired a specialty physician, $10,000 for a primary-care physician, $7,000 for a nurse practitioner or physician assistant, $5,000 for a nurse. This would also serve as an incentive to hire the type of worker who could provide the most cost-effective care. Right now, employers are paying $15,000 to $25,000 to recruit just one healthcare worker from abroad. That money could be used to help train a nurse in this country. Another option would be to ask health insurers to pay $10 per year per person enrolled in their insurance programs, public and private, to contribute toward training new health workers. With our current insurance coverage rates, that would generate $2.6 billion per year for additional health-worker training. If we were to achieve full insurance coverage, $3 billion per year would be generated.

Open the Federal Bonding System to All Funders

While community-based recruitment and training are the best ways by far to ensure that healthcare workers practice in underserved communities, bonding systems can have a positive—if temporary—effect. As I explained earlier, bonding, or return service, is a good way to help students pay for their education. It can also affect where healthcare workers practice, at least for a few years. In return for a scholarship from the bonding organization, students agree to enter a primary-care field after graduation and to practice in an underserved community for a certain number of years. If the student does not fulfill the agreement, he or she has to repay the scholarship money.

Bonding is not mandatory. Students who are not interested in a bonding contract still have unrestricted federal student loans available to them. Those who do sign a contract can break it at any time, on the condition that they repay the money over a reasonable period of time.

Bonding does require a sophisticated administrative system, to verify that healthcare workers are practicing in the communities they are supposed to and to provide legal clout when a contract has been violated. The largest federal healthcare-worker bonding program is the National Health Service Corps, which bonds students to practice primary care in underserved communities. At present, bonding occurs only at the federal level, with federal money, but there is no real reason for that limitation. Any funder—whether a state, a county, a community, a foundation, a charity, or an individual—should be able to participate in the bonding system.

Let's say a church in rural Alabama wants to help the community gain another nurse. The church might raise $30,000 to pay for tuition in a three-year associate-RN program and, in return, require the graduating student to work in primary care anywhere in the church's home county for six years (two years for each year of the scholarship). The church could decide whether the scholarship would be tied to a particular nursing school, presumably near the church, or could be used in any nursing school. It would contact the National Health Service Corps scholarship program to let it know the amount of the scholarship and the bonding terms (community and number of years of service) and pay the school directly. The corps would provide a standard contract and monitor the compliance of both parties. If the person who received the scholarship did not meet her obligation—if she left the community after just three years of service, say—the corps would be responsible for ensuring that she paid the church back.

It's not too much to say that allowing more organizations to pay into the federal bonding program could revolutionize the funding of healthcare-worker education in this country.

Increase Healthcare Workers' Productivity

Inefficient use of healthcare workers greatly exacerbates the healthcare-worker shortage. If we could increase the productivity of the healthcare workers we have—and keep more of them from dropping out altogether—we would significantly reduce the number of workers we need to train and employ in the future.

Productivity can be increased in a variety of ways. For one thing, we really need to modernize and streamline the way healthcare facilities work. McDonald's thinks much more about the efficiency of its operations than most hospitals do, including for-profit hospitals. Hospitals and clinics have a lot to learn from private businesses in other sectors. The healthcare sector has been very quick to adopt clinical innovations, such as the latest cancer drug or the da Vinci remote surgical system. But it has been glacially slow in adopting management systems and information technology that would increase the efficiency of healthcare staff; most healthcare organizations have yet to adopt the most basic efficiency and systems innovations.

For example, although electronic medical records have been available since the 1960s, the office staff of most physicians' offices still use incredibly inefficient paper-based recordkeeping. In addition, most people who supervise other healthcare workers have little or no management or supervisory training, so they're usually unable to help the staff be as productive as it could be. If hospitals and clinics focused on identifying tasks that can be eliminated, simplified, or delegated to a more appropriate type of worker, it would save countless person-hours as well as countless sums of money in the long run.

Better division of labor can result in more cost-effective and higher-quality care. Someone with as many years of higher education as a registered nurse should not be changing bedpans; a properly trained licensed practical nurse or nurse's aide can do this task. The vast majority of primary-care patients can be cared for by nurse practitioners, physician assistants, and advanced-practice nurses. Physicians, particularly subspecialists, should practice at the top of their licenses; they should care for only the sickest patients and those with less common or hard-to-manage diseases.

The healthcare sector has higher rates of early retirement and labor-market dropout (that is, choosing not to work in that field anymore) than many industries. Much of the early retirement is due to the higher wages that healthcare workers are paid; when you make more than twice the national annual salary, it's financially feasible to retire earlier. But there are other reasons for dropout and early retirement. Burnout is a problem.[11]

Despite the extremely high rewards, the work is often stressful; lives are at stake. In addition to worrying about the health of their patients, healthcare providers are concerned about increased direct exposure to infections such as tuberculosis, HIV, hepatitis C, and epidemic influenza. By providing easily accessible stress-reduction programs, we can help healthcare workers better manage the inherent stress of their jobs. We need to provide more supportive and less bureaucratic working environments, too.

Many female healthcare workers, as well as retired healthcare workers of both sexes, would reenter the workforce if they could have flexible schedules. Offering shifts of, say, nine hours rather than 12 hours would help healthcare workers who have family responsibilities. In its 80-plus centers, the Cleveland Clinic, world famous for the quality of its care, offers its nurses "parent shifts" that last from two to six hours.[12] In Nashville, Vanderbilt University Medical Center has a web-based system that allows nurses to schedule their shifts online. This gives them more control over their schedules than the traditional method: sending their manager their shift preferences and then being forced to work whatever shifts they are assigned.

The clinic where I work has done an excellent job of making work more flexible and family friendly. Some of the physicians work only four days a week, and an electronic medical-record system allows the doctors to complete their notes, check lab results, and design treatment plans from home. For the convenience of patients, the clinic offers weekend hours, but regular pediatricians don't always have to work them. Instead, the clinic hires part-timers like me.

In addition, to keep many younger and retirement-age healthcare workers employed, it is important to offer part-time work. Part-time work presents a particular challenge to physicians, whose malpractice-insurance rates are orders of magnitude higher than for any other type of healthcare worker. Many non-working younger physicians and retired older physicians would like to work a few hours a week or month but can't afford the malpractice insurance. Most malpractice insurers charge the same amount whether a physician works 10 or 80 hours a week. Requiring malpractice insurers to charge physicians per hours worked rather than a flat rate would enable thousands of physicians to reenter the workforce part-time.

Rationalize the US Healthcare Labor Market

The training and placement of healthcare workers, and the incentive systems to retain them in underserved areas, is a patchwork of self-interested solutions and Band-Aid fixes. No one entity coordinates the most valuable part of the US healthcare system: the workforce. With thousands of commissions, boards, and schools determining how many and what type of healthcare workers are produced each year, it's no wonder we do not have the workforce we need.

It would not take a Soviet-style central-planning regulatory body to oversee and coordinate the process. I would like to see the Department of Health and Human Services, particularly the Health Resources and Services Administration and its Bureau of Health Professions, take on this role. The Bureau of Health Professions could start the process by collecting and analyzing the data on the education costs, annual number of graduates, and scope of practice decisions for each type of healthcare worker.

We have an incredible opportunity in that the recent health

reform created a National Health Workforce Commission. For the first time, there is an organization tasked with making recommendations to Congress, the Department of Health and Human Services, and the Department of Labor on how to address the national healthcare-worker shortage. The membership of the commission consists of representatives from schools, insurers, hospital systems, and unions, as well as health-workforce experts. Working with the Bureau of Health Professions, the commission can take a nonpartisan look at the healthcare workforce and consider what is best not for individual healthcare professions or companies but for the American people and the healthcare system as a whole.

But the National Health Workforce Commission has not yet been funded by Congress and therefore cannot meet. I argue that this would be a small but significant investment toward reaching workforce self-sufficiency in the largest sector of our economy.

Mitigate the Impact of the Recruitment of Foreign Healthcare Workers

The United States cannot end its dependence on imported healthcare workers overnight. It will take at least a decade to achieve this goal. In the meantime, we can take measures to reduce the negative impact—at home and abroad—of bringing so many healthcare workers here from developing countries.

Because the practice of recruiting foreign healthcare workers is rife with abuses, many international and US healthcare organizations already support industry regulation. These include the American Hospital Association; the National Council of State Nursing Boards; the Service Employees International Union (SEIU, the country's largest healthcare-worker union); the International Council of Nurses (which represents more than 130 national nurses' associations); and the World Health Organization.[13] The recruitment industry itself supports regulation and has even formed an industry group, the American Association of International Healthcare Recruitment.

Once again, I am not proposing new agencies. What I would like to see is all the organizations involved in recruiting and hiring foreign healthcare workers collaborating under the auspices of an existing agency, whose highest interest is the American people and economy rather than a single profession or hospital system. Most likely, that agency would be the Bureau of Health Professions.

At present, there is no regulation of the companies that recruit foreign healthcare workers. The Joint Commission—a global, nongovernmental organization that rates the quality of care in hospitals and other health-services organizations—has a voluntary certification program for healthcare-staffing agencies. For the purposes of certification, quality is analyzed through various objective measures, such as the percentage of placements in which the staff member is requested not to return to the facility (for either clinical or professional misbehavior) and the percentage of staff that has attended some type of orientation, in, say, cultural knowledge or infection control. Medicare and other health insurers use the Joint Commission's hospital certification to determine whether they will pay for care at that hospital. It would be quite consistent with existing policy for Medicare to require Joint Commission certification of staffing agencies as well. A large percentage of foreign-trained nurses enter the United States through these agencies. This would be a convenient way to ensure that these nurses receive appropriate orientation to US practice standards and that their quality of care is monitored.

There is a nonbinding, voluntary code of conduct for nurse recruitment; it does not go far enough to protect nurses from abuse by recruiters or to protect the health of their patients. The majority of the code focuses on complying with fundamental US labor laws, such as not discriminating when hiring based on age or sex or national origin. Other parts of the code cover not providing false or misleading information and complying with the laws of the nurse's country of origin—pretty basic stuff.[14]

We can make better use of these mechanisms, but we need to go further. The Bureau of Health Professions should work with the recruiting companies to develop binding rules on how they function in the United States and abroad. Recruiting companies should no longer be allowed to set up tables at graduation ceremonies or otherwise recruit through health-professional schools. They should not be able to recruit through professional associations, such as nurse or physician unions or councils, their staff, events, job fairs, or publications. Recruiting could continue through non-healthcare-specific media, such as the Internet or local telephone books.

The contract process must also be improved. As discussed in chapter 3, many foreign-trained nurses working in the United States are subject to extremely high fees if they choose to break their contract with the recruitment agency, whether to work for another agency or to return home. This effectively makes them indentured servants. Such contract-buyout fees should be eliminated or, at the very least, limited to the original investment the company made in the worker. If buyout fees remain, the payback process should be regulated so that the foreign healthcare worker has a reasonable period in which to make the payments.

There should be a grievance process in place that allows foreign healthcare workers to report problems without fearing deportation or other retaliation. Workers will never report problems or abuse unless they know they will be free from harassment during the investigation.

When foreign healthcare workers arrive in this country, they should be required to attend a standard orientation course to introduce them to the US healthcare system. This course could be provided by their recruiting agency or the health facility, but it would follow a standard curriculum for each healthcare profession. The course would cover the roles and responsibilities of each member of the healthcare team, as well as cultural issues that affect quality of care in the United States. The course would review the most common diagnoses and treatments for the patient population the foreign healthcare provider will be working with and offer training in the relevant equipment and procedures. For instance, a foreign-trained nurse preparing to work in a pediatric hospital would review or learn the most common diagnoses, treatments, and procedures for hospitalized children (including asthma, fever in infants, and pneumonia), as well as how to handle the relevant equipment. Newly arrived healthcare workers should be matched with an experienced US worker in their workplace, who would serve as a mentor for at least one year.

Perhaps most important, we should immediately change the nature of the visas offered foreign healthcare workers: All such visas should be specifically limited to four or five years. When the visa expires, the worker must leave the United States. Healthcare facilities should not be allowed to hire workers with expired visas, nor should state licensing boards renew the licenses of healthcare workers on expired visas. Enforcement of these new rules should be through existing enforcement channels.

We should definitely address the fact that importing healthcare workers hurts some countries more than others. Bringing one physician to the United States from India denies that country 0.0001 percent of its physicians. Bringing just one physician to the United States from Liberia denies that country 1 percent of its physicians. Both countries have shortages and maldistributions of healthcare workers, but far more damage is done when we take healthcare workers from the countries that need their healthcare workers most.

We need to make certain that we give no healthcare-worker visas to doctors and nurses who have not fulfilled their service requirements in their own countries. Most healthcare workers in developing countries are trained with public funds, and many governments require them to practice medicine in that country for a specified number of years. The United States does not check to see whether those who apply for its special healthcare-worker visas have satisfied this obligation. It should not be difficult to begin doing so. Once a year, the countries that have service requirements for their healthcare workers could send the State Department—the agency that processes all visas—a list of the workers who have not yet fulfilled those requirements. The State Department would check the names of visa applicants against this list; it could ask those whose names are on the list to reapply when they have fulfilled their legal obligations.

We should designate countries with the most acute healthcare-worker shortages as "no hit" countries for healthcare-worker visas. Healthcare workers from these countries would remain eligible for lottery, family, refugee, and vacation visas; their immigration rights would not be violated. We simply would make them ineligible for earmarked healthcare work visas. Until then, we could place a cap on the number of visas issued each year to healthcare workers from those countries. The caps could be phased in gradually, to give the new US-based training programs I've recommended time to produce more American workers, and to give the recruiting companies a chance to find alternative sources of recruits.

As noted in chapter 4, healthcare workers who travel from developing countries to developed countries usually do not return home. When they do, the knowledge they have gained is rarely applicable and can even be damaging, because they have learned to rely on expensive, technology-dependent forms of diagnosis and treatment that increase costs without a commensurate improvement in outcomes, if they are even available in their home countries.

What I am suggesting offers a chance to make the myth of "cycled migration" a reality. Truly circular healthcare-worker migration would work as follows. Moving forward, all new healthcare-worker visas would be temporary, without an option for extension. While in this country, these workers would be in the type of facility with which they have the most experience: If they work in a healthcare clinic in their own country, they would work in a healthcare clinic in the United States; if they work in a hospital at home, they would work in a hospital here. Only senior healthcare workers would be eligible for healthcare-worker visas—not only because of their more extensive knowledge and experience, but also because they would have the clout to influence their practice areas when they return home.

While working in the American hospital or clinic, foreign healthcare workers should be given a project relevant to a challenge in their home institutions. A nurse from a Jamaican hospital plagued with hospital-acquired infections could focus on learning how her American hospital prevents infections. A Tanzanian physician whose clinic has difficulty getting tuberculosis patients to comply with their medication schedules would learn how his American clinic deals with that kind of problem. Or they could focus on how health facilities are managed, a skill that more readily translates to low-resource settings.

Ideally, cycled migration would involve the home-country employers of the healthcare workers, so that they could return to the same facility. While in the United States, they would maintain contact with their home facility to ensure that the project they are working on here remains relevant to their country's needs. On returning, they could help their former healthcare facilities on the issue they studied while in this country.

Another way to manage migration is for recruiters or healthcare facilities that hire foreign-trained workers for their first jobs in this country to pay for the cost of their education. Already some recruiters have expressed a willingness to do this if all recruiters participate. The payments could go to the school itself or to the Ministry of Health or Ministry of Education that oversees the school. This would enable the country to pay for the education of replacement healthcare workers. The payment should cover only the cost of the worker's education; it should not be a source of profit. Otherwise, the schools might abandon their mandate to train healthcare workers for the domestic market in favor of the profit-making American market.

If this book has raised concerns for you regarding how we train health workers in the United States and insource those from other countries, please contact your local health-professional school or community college. Work with them to start and expand programs to invest in people from your community and fill jobs in your community. Let your local, state, and national representatives know that this is an issue that matters to you and your family.

The pedestal on the Statue of Liberty is inscribed with the famous lines "Give me your tired, your poor, your huddled masses yearning to breathe free." We have abandoned these values for something along the lines of "Give me the cream of your crop, leaving you unable to care for your own people." In its unofficial policy toward the training of healthcare workers, the United

States has moved far from its own values and has abandoned its own young people in the process. It's time we lived up to those values. It's time we addressed our health-workforce challenges with American solutions.

Notes

Introduction

1 Organization for Economic Cooperation and Development, *Immigrant Health Workers in OECD Countries in the Broader Context of Highly Skilled Migration* (Paris: OECD, 2007), 165; "OECD Statistical Extracts," OECD, accessed November 4, 2008, at http://stats.oecd.org/Index.aspx.

2 Louisa Lim, "Is Trade War Brewing over Chinese Tire Imports?" NPR, September 22, 2009, www.npr.org/templates/story/story.php?storyId=113052532.

3 Yu Xu, "Are Chinese Nurses a Viable Source for the Nursing Shortage?," *Nursing Economics* 21, no. 6 (2003).

4 Adam Davidson, "World Sock Capital Suffers from Duty-Free Imports," NPR, November 10, 2009, www.npr.org/templates/story/story.php?storyId=16661333.

5 "Health Care Worker Visas," American Visa Bureau, accessed January 15, 2009, at www.visabureau.com/america/health-care.aspx.

6 J. Needleman et al., "Nurse Staffing and Inpatient Hospital Mortality," *New England Journal of Medicine* 364, no. 11 (March 17, 2011): 1037–45; A. M. Trinkoff et al., "Nurses' Work Schedule Characteristics, Nurse Staffing, and Patient Mortality," *Nursing Research* 60, no. 1 (January-February 2011): 1–8; P. F. Pronovost et al., "Physician Staffing Patterns and Clinical Outcomes in Critically Ill Patients: A Systematic Review," *Journal of the American Medical Association* 288, no. 17 (November 6, 2002): 2151–62.

7 B. L. Brush, J. Sochalski, and A. M. Berger, "Imported Care: Recruiting Foreign Nurses to U.S. Health Care Facilities," *Health Affairs* 23, no. 3 (2004): 78–87.

8 Nancy Chege and Maryanne Garon, "Adaptation Challenges Facing Internationally Educated Nurses," *Dimensions of Critical Care Nursing* 29, no. 3 (May/June 2010): 131–35; Yu Xu, "Communicative

Competence of International Nurses and Patient Safety and Quality of Care," *Home HealthCare Management and Practice* 20, no. 5 (2008): 430–32.

9 Agency for Healthcare Research and Quality, *National Healthcare Disparities Report* (Washington, DC: AHRQ, 2010).

10 "Racial Health Disparities by the Numbers," Center for American Progress, accessed February 2, 2010, at www.americanprogress.org/issues/2010/01/health_disparity_numbers.html.

11 Association of American Medical Colleges, *Medical School Debt* (Washington, DC: AAMC, 2009).

12 American Association of Nursing Colleges, *Alleviate the Nursing Faculty Shortage: Support the Nurses' Higher Education and Loan Repayment (HEAL) Act* (Washington, DC: AANC, 2009).

13 Gregory A. Smith, *Attitudes toward Immigration: In the Pulpit and the Pew* (Washington, DC: Pew Charitable Trust, 2006).

14 "OECD Statistical Extracts," OECD, accessed November 4, 2008, at http://stats.oecd.org/Index.aspx.

Chapter 1. Shortage in the Land of Abundance

1 "National Health Expenditure Data: NHE Fact Sheet," Centers for Medicare and Medicaid Services (CMS), accessed September 16, 2009, at www.cms.gov/NationalHealthExpendData/25_NHE_Fact_Sheet.asp. Sean Keehan et al., "Health Spending Projections through 2017: The Baby-Boom Generation Is Coming to Medicare," *Health Affairs* Web Exclusive, February 26, 2008, content.healthaffairs.org/content/27/2/w145.abstract.

2 "CMS National Health Expenditure Projections 2009–2019," CMS, accessed September 17, 2009, at www.cms.hhs.gov/NationalHealthExpendData/downloads/proj2009.pdf. Debra Wood, "Nursing Jobs Grow Despite Recession," Nurse Zone, accessed September 17, 2009, at www.nursezone.com/Nursing-News-Events/more-news/Nursing-Jobs-Grow-Despite-Recession_28286.aspx.

3 Associated Press, "Woman Dies in ER Lobby," MSNBC, June 13, 2007, www.msnbc.msn.com/id/19207050/ns/health-health_care/t/woman-dies-er-lobby-refuses-help/.

4 Phyllis Greene, "The Cases of Negligence Due to Nurse Understaffing," eHow Health, accessed September 17, 2009, at www.ehow.com/about_5668945_cases-negligence-due-nurse-understaffing.html.

5 Institute of Medicine, "To Err Is Human: Building a Safer Health System," November 1, 1999, www.iom.edu/~/media/Files/Report%20Files/1999/To-Err-is-Human/To%20Err%20is%20Human%201999%20%20report%20brief.pdf.

6 Linda Aikin et al., "Hospital Nurse Staffing and Patient Mortality, Nurse Burnout, and Job Dissatisfaction," *Journal of the American Medical Association* 288, no. 16 (2002): 1987–93.

7 Joint Commission on Accreditation of Healthcare Organizations, *Health Care at the Crossroads: Strategies for Addressing the Evolving Nursing Crisis* (Washington, DC: JCAHO, 2009).

8 Deanna Bellandi, "Number of Patients per Nurse: Life/Death," Associated Press, October 22, 2002.

9 Anita Catlin, "Pediatric Medical Errors, Part 2: Case Commentary, a Source of Tremendous Loss," *Pediatric Nursing* 30, no. 4 (2004): 331–35.

10 R. Blendon et al., "Views of Practicing Physicians and the Public on Medical Errors," *New England Journal of Medicine* 347, no. 24 (December 12, 2002): 1933–40.

11 "Palomar Pomerado Health Reports Significant Drop in Turnover Rate," *Knight Ridder/Tribune Business News*, February 10, 2005.

12 CMS, *Minimum Nurse Staffing Ratios in Nursing Homes* (Washington, DC: CMS, 2002).

13 Robert Lowes, "Largest Ever Nurses' Strike Could Be Sign of Future Unrest," *Medscape Medical News*, June 11, 2010.

14 Health Resources and Services Administration, *The Physician Workforce: Projections and Research into Current Issues Affecting Supply and Demand* (Washington, DC: HRSA, 2008).

15 "Doctor Dearth: Frustrated with Managed Care and Flush with Wise Investment, Physicians Are Retiring Earlier—Alarming Hospitals and Practices," *Hospitals & Health Networks* 75, no. 3 (2001).

16 "U.S. Physician Shortage Particularly Affects Rural Hospitals," *Medical News Today*, February 27, 2008.

17 "OECD Database," OECD, accessed November 1, 2010, at www.oecd.org/dataoecd/53/12/38976551.pdf.

18 Alan Porter, "Primary Physician Shortage Spurs Search for Alternatives," *Examiner*, August 24, 2009, www.examiner.com/x-5968-DC-Public-Policy-Examiner~y2009m8d24-Physician-shortage-spurs-search-for-alternatives.

19 Richard Dehn, "Physician Shortage Predictions and Their Implications," *Journal of American Academy of Physician Assistants*, July 1, 2008, www.jaapa.com/physician-shortage-predictions-and-their-implications/article/124085/.

20 "Physician Shortages to Worsen without Increases in Residency Training," Association of American Medical Schools, accessed July 5, 2010, at www.aamc.org/download/150612/data/md-shortage.pdf.

21 Mark D. Schwartz et al., "Changes in Medical Students' Views of Internal Medicine Careers from 1990 to 2007," *Archives of Internal Medicine* 171, no. 8 (2011): 744–49, doi:10.1001/archinternmed.2011.139.

22 Douglas Staiger, David Auerbach, and Peter Buerhaus, "Trends in the Work Hours of Physicians in the United States," *Journal of the American Medical Association* 303 (2010): 747–53.

23 "Nursing by the Numbers Fact Sheet," American Nursing Association, accessed October 10, 2009, at www.nursingworld.org/NursingbytheNumbersFactSheet.aspx.

24 "Nursing Workforce Projections," HRSA, Bureau of Health Professions, accessed November 1, 2010, at http://bhpr.hrsa.gov/healthworkforce/reports/behindrnprojections/2.htm.

25 Claire Brocato, "Wisdom at Work: Success Strategies for Keeping Your Most Experienced Nurses," AMN Healthcare, accessed June 1, 2009, at http://amnhealthcare.com/News/news-details.aspx?Id=32272.

26 Bernard Hodes Group, "Aging Nursing Workforce Study," accessed June 1, 2009, at www.hodes.com/resources/library/researchreports/aging-nursing-workforce-study.

27 "Nursing Shortage Fact Sheet," AACN, accessed June 3, 2009, at www.aacn.nche.edu/Media/FactSheets/NursingShortage.htm.

28 Patricia Pittman, Amanda Folsom, Emily Bass, and Kathryn

Leonhardy, *U.S.-Based International Nurse Recruitment: Structure and Practices of a Burgeoning Industry* (Washington, DC: Academy Health, 2007).

29 "California Suffers from Severe Nurse Shortage," Online Nursing School Guys, accessed July 11, 2009, at www.online-nursing-school-guys.com/articles/california_understaffed.php.

30 "Nursing Shortage Fact Sheet," AACN, accessed June 3, 2009, at www.aacn.nche.edu/Media/FactSheets/NursingShortage.htm.

31 S. Pal, "Pharmacist Shortage to Worsen in 2020," *U.S. Pharmacist* 27, no. 12 (2002); Association of Colleges of Pharmacy, "Dramatic Rise in Need for Pharmacists Projected," accessed November 2, 2010, at www.aacp.org/site/tertiary.asp?TRACKID=&VID=2&CID=577&DID=4638. Jennifer Larson, "Other Health Care Personnel Shortages Affect Nurses, Patient Care," *Nursing Zone* (2002), accessed September 30, 2009, at www.nursezone.com/nursing-news-events/more-news/Other-Health-Care-Personnel-Shortages-Affect-Nurses-Patient-Care_28426.aspx.

32 "Retail Prescription Drugs Filled at Pharmacies," Kaiser Foundation, accessed November 2, 2010, at www.statehealthfacts.org/comparetable.jsp?ind=268&cat=5.

33 "Hepatitis A Outbreak Associated with Green Onions at a Restaurant—Monaca, Pennsylvania, 2003," *Morbidity and Mortality Weekly Report* 52, no. 47 (November 28, 2003): 1155–57, www.cdc.gov/mmwr/preview/mmwrhtml/mm5247a5.htm.

34 "The Registered Nurse Population: Findings from the 2008 National Sample Survey of Registered Nurses," US HHS Bureau for Health Professions Research, accessed September 1, 2009, at http://bhpr.hrsa.gov/healthworkforce/.

35 "HealthSouth Rehabilitation Hospital FAQS," HealthSouth, accessed November 7, 2010, at www.infoimagination.org/test/healthsouthnm/faqs.html.

36 K. Burns et al., "Increasing Prevalence of Medically Complex Children in US Hospitals," *Pediatrics* 126, no. 4 (October 2010): 638–46.

37 "Overweight and Obesity Trends among Adults," CDC, accessed November 7, 2010, at www.cdc.gov/obesity/data/index.html.

38 "AAMC: Health Reform Law to Exacerbate Doctor Shortage,"

California Healthline, accessed October 4, 2011, at www.californiahealthline.org/articles/2010/10/4/aamc-health-reform-law-to-exacerbate-doctor-shortage.aspx.

39 "Physician Shortages to Worsen without Increases in Residency Training," Association of American Medical Schools, accessed July 5, 2010, at www.aamc.org/download/150612/data/md-shortage.pdf.

40 "Seton Releases Study Showing Physician Shortage Hitting Close to Home," Seton Hospitals, accessed October 2, 2009, at www.seton.net/about_seton/news/2009/03/25/seton_releases_study_showing_physician_shortage_hitting_close_to_home.

41 "Doctor Dearth: Frustrated with Managed Care and Flush with Wise Investment, Physicians Are Retiring Earlier—Alarming Hospitals and Practices," *Hospitals & Health Networks* 75, no. 3 (March 2001), accessed September 1, 2009, at www.nejmjobs.org/rpt/early-retirement-physicians.aspx.

42 Dave Taylor, "Study Confirms Wabash Valley Health Care Worker Shortage," Indiana State University, April 1, 2010, www.indstate.edu/news/news.php?newsid=2181.

43 Carol Adaire Jones et al., *Health Status and Health Care Access of Farm and Rural Populations* (Washington, DC: USDA, 2009).

44 Liz Kowalczyk, "Waits to See Hub Doctors Grow Longer, Busiest Practices Have No Openings for a Year," *Boston Globe*, May 15, 2009, www.boston.com/news/health/articles/2009/05/15/waits_to_see_hub_doctors_grow_longer/.

45 *2009 Survey of Physician Appointment Wait Times* (Irving, TX: Merritt Hawkins, 2009), accessed September 11, 2009, at www.merritthawkins.com/pdf/mha2009waittimesurvey.pdf. D. O. Straiger et al., "Trends in the Work Hours of Physicians in the United States," *Journal of the American Medical Association* 303 (2010): 747–53.

46 A. Guttmann, "Primary Care Physician Supply and Children's Health Care Use, Access, and Outcomes: Findings from Canada," *Pediatrics* 125, no. 6 (June 2010): 1119–26.

47 Ibid.

48 "California Feels Nurse Anesthetists' Pinch," Encyclopedia.com, accessed September 30, 2009, at www.encyclopedia.com/doc/1G1-126016387.html.

49 Richard Cooper, personal communication with the author, November 28, 2009.

Chapter 2. How the United States Created Its Healthcare-Workforce Problem

1 Bureau of Labor Statistics, "Career Guide to Industries, 2010–11 Edition: Healthcare," accessed October 1, 2009, at www.bls.gov/oco/cg/cgs035.htm.

2 "U.S. Medical School Applicants and Students," Association of American Medical Schools, accessed December 20, 2010, at www.aamc.org/download/153708/data/charts1982to2011.pdf.

3 B. Bernstein and B. Ensminger, "It's Time to Fund Physician Shortage Programs by Abandoning Unrestricted State Subsidies to Medical Schools," *Journal of Health Politics, Policy and Law* 8, no. 2 (1983): 221–34.

4 *Medical School Tuition and Young Physician Indebtedness* (Washington, DC: Association of American Medical Schools, 2007).

5 Praveen Ghanta, "US Doctors Are Overeducated," July 2, 2009, http://truecostblog.com/2009/07/02/us-doctors-are-overeducated/.

6 Andrew H. Beck, "The Flexner Report and the Standardization of American Medical Education," *Journal of the American Medical Association* 291 (2004): 2139–40, http://jama.ama-assn.org/cgi/content/full/291/17/2139.

7 Ibid.

8 Ibid.

9 Esther Brown, *Nursing for the Future* (Princeton, NJ: Carnegie Foundation, 1948).

10 "Is the Nursing Shortage Affecting HealthCare?," ArticlesBase, July 20, 2009, www.articlesbase.com/health-articles/is-the-nursing-shortage-affecting-healthcare-1053485.html.

11 "The Doctor of Nursing Practice Fact Sheet," American Association of Colleges of Nursing, accessed September 22, 2010, at www.aacn.nche.edu/Media/FactSheets/dnp.htm.

12 Institute of Medicine, "To Err Is Human: Building a Safer Health System," November 1, 1999, www.iom.edu/~/media/Files/Report

%20Files/1999/To-Err-is-Human/To%20Err%20is%20Human %201999%20%20report%20brief.pdf. Quote: p. 2.

13 W. McGaghie, "Perspectives on Medical School Admissions," *Academic Medicine* 65, no. 3 (March 1990): 136–39.

14 C. Elam and M. Johnson, "Prediction of Medical Students' Academic Performances: Does the Admission Interview Help?," *Academic Medicine* 67 (1992): S28–S30.

15 M. Hojat et al., "Students' Psychosocial Characteristics as Predictors of Academic Performance in Medical School," *Academic Medicine* 68 (1993): 635–37.

16 "What Are the Qualities of a Good Physician?," Medicine World, accessed September 2, 2010, at http://medicineworld.org/cancer/lead/3-2006/what-are-the-qualities-of-a-good-physician.html.

17 "LCME Members, 2010–2011," Liaison Committee on Medical Education, accessed November 21, 2010, at www.lcme.org/members.htm.

18 "Tuition Inflation," FinAid, accessed November 27, 2009, at www.finaid.org/savings/tuition-inflation.phtml.

Chapter 3. The Path to America

1 "Match Press Release," AAMC, accessed June 27, 2010, at www.aamc.org/newsroom/pressrel/2010/100318.htm.

2 G. McMahon, "Coming to America—International Medical Graduates in the United States," *New England Journal of Medicine* 350, no. 24 (June 10, 2004): 2435–37; E. Akl et al., "The United States Physician Workforce and International Medical Graduates: Trends and Characteristics," *Journal of General Internal Medicine* 22, no. 2 (2007): 264–68.

3 "NCLEX," National Council of State Boards of Nursing, February 12, 2004, www.ncsbn.org/research_stats/nclex.asp.

4 B. L. Brush, J. Sochalski, and A. M. Berger, "Imported Care: Recruiting Foreign Nurses to U.S. Health Care Facilities," *Health Affairs* 23, no. 3 (2004): 78–87.

5 "Need Help Getting a US Residency," Craigslist, accessed August 24, 2009, at http://chicago.craigslist.org/nch/hea/1322437529.html.

6 "FMG America: A Possible Fraud?," IMG Digest, accessed November 26, 2010, at www.usmletomd.com/imgdigest/2007/11/fmgamerica-possible-fraud.html.

7 "Be Careful with Fraud Residency Programs," Residency Forum, March 31, 2008, www.residencyforum.com/viewtopic.php?t=5929.

8 Barbara Bein, "IMGs Seeking Positions in U.S. Residencies Now Can Join ECFMG Advice Network," American Academy of Family Practice, June 17, 2010, www.aafp.org/online/en/home/publications/news/news-now/resident-student-focus/20100617imgnetwork.html.

9 IMG Digest, accessed August 24, 2009, at www.usmletomd.com/imgdigest/.

10 David Rose, "Foreign Doctors Face Competence Inquiry," *Sunday Times* (London), August 10, 2007.

11 "Doctor Sued for Fake Diagnosis," ABC News, June 15, 2010, www.wxyz.com/dpp/news/local_news/doctor-sued-for-fake-diagnosis.

12 P. Pittman et al., *U.S.-Based International Nurse Recruitment: Structure and Practices of a Burgeoning Industry* (Washington, DC: Academy Health, 2007).

13 Ibid.

14 Ibid.

15 Ibid.

16 *Business Week* Stock Database, Business Week, accessed November 1, 2009, at www.businessweek.com/investor/stocks/.

17 "Ethical Nurse Recruitment Position Statement," ICN, accessed July 21, 2009, at www.icn.ch/psrecruit01.htm.

18 P. Pittman et al., *U.S.-Based International Nurse Recruitment: Structure and Practices of a Burgeoning Industry* (Washington, DC: Academy Health, 2007).

19 Ibid.

20 Joseph Lariosa, "Filipino Nurses Win vs Sentosa in NY Court," GMANews, May 30, 2010, www.gmanews.tv/story/192219/filipino-nurses-win-vs-sentosa-in-ny-court.

21 Pittman et al., *U.S.-Based International Nurse Recruitment*.

22 "Military Accessions Vital to National Interest (MAVNI) Recruitment Pilot," Department of Defense, accessed September 10, 2009, at www.defense.gov/news/mavni-fact-sheet.pdf.

23 Matt Richtel, "Tech Recruiting Clashes with Immigration Rules," *New York Times*, April 11, 2009, www.nytimes.com/2009/04/12/business/12immig.html?_r=1&th=&emc=th&pagewanted=all.

24 "Exchange Visitor Visas," Department of State, accessed November 17, 2010, at travel.state.gov/visa/temp/types/types_1267.html.

25 "J-1 Visa Waivers," GovTrack.us, accessed September 24, 2009, at www.govtrack.us/congress/record.xpd?id=110-h20071218-4.

26 Ibid.

27 Ibid.

Chapter 4. The Damage Done

1 "Ethiopia Country Statistics," UNICEF, accessed September 24, 2009, at www.unicef.org/infobycountry/ethiopia_statistics.html.

2 Caglar Ozden et al., "Patterns of Migration in Ghanaian Nurses and Physicians," World Bank, unpublished, 2009.

3 "Human Resource Shortage Affecting Rural Health Mission: PM," NewKerala.com, November 3, 2009, www.newkerala.com/nkfullnews-1-143111.html.

4 World Health Organization, *Working Together for Health: World Health Report* (Geneva: WHO, 2006).

5 L. Chen et al., *Human Resources for Health: Overcoming the Crisis* (Cambridge, MA: Harvard University Press, 2004).

6 Anja Schoepes et al., "The Effect of Distance to Health-Care Facilities on Childhood Mortality in Rural Burkina Faso," *American Journal of Epidemiology* 173, no. 5 (2011): 492–98.

7 S. Anand and T. Bärnighausen, "Health Workers and Vaccination Coverage in Developing Countries: An Econometric Analysis," *Lancet* 369, no. 9569 (April 14, 2007): 1277–85.

8 M. Tuoane, N. Madise, and I. Diamond, "Provision of Family Planning Services in Lesotho," *International Family Planning Perspectives* 30, no. 2 (June 2004), accessed July 21, 2009, at www.jstor.org/pss/3181030.

9 "Health Action in Crises: Lesotho," World Health Organization, last modified September 2005, accessed July 21, 2009, at www.who.int/hac/crises/lso/background/Lesotho_aug05_rev.pdf.

10 Alex Preker, Director, Health in Africa Initiative, International Finance Corporation, personal communication to author, September 23, 2010.

11 Amy Hagopian, Associate Professor, University of Washington School of Public Health, personal communication to author, March 23, 2010.

12 ECFMG, "Medical School Accreditation Requirement for ECFMG Certification," last updated September 21, 2010, accessed September 21, 2010, at www.ecfmg.org/accreditation.

13 Note: Underemployed people either do not have full-time jobs or have jobs that do not provide them with a living wage.

14 Joses Kirigia et al., "The Cost of Health Professionals' Brain Drain in Kenya," *BMC Health Services Research* 6, no. 89 (2006): 1–10.

15 A. S. Muula and B. Panulo, "Lost Investment Returns from the Migration of Medical Doctors from Malawi," *Tanzanian Health Research Bulletin* 9, no. 1 (January 2007): 61–64.

16 Stephen Ohlemacher, "Number of Illegal Immigrants Hits 12M," Associated Press, March 7, 2006, www.breitbart.com/article.php?id=D8G6u2ko8&show_article=1.

17 D. G. Kassebaum et al., "On Rising Medical Student Debt: In for a Penny, In for a Pound," *Academic Medicine* 71, no. 10 (October 1996): 1124–34; M. Valcarcel, C. Diaz, and P. J. Santiago-Borrero, "Training and Retaining of Underrepresented Minority Physician Scientists—a Hispanic Perspective: NICHD-AAP Workshop on Research in Neonatology," *Journal of Perinatology* 26, suppl. 2 (July 2006): S49–S52.

18 "UN Security Council on AIDS in Africa," Encyclopedia Britannica, accessed May 31, 2010, at www.britannica.com/bps/additionalcontent/18/8860103/UN-Security-Council-Session-on-AIDS-in-Africa.

19 Jennifer Epstein, "George W. Bush Urges Congress to Fight AIDS," *Politico*, December 1, 2010, www.politico.com/news/stories/1210/45793.html.

20 "Obama's National Security Strategy Released, Includes Global Health, Food Security Priorities," Kaiser Daily Global Health Policy Report, May 31, 2010, www.medicalnewstoday.com/articles/190354.php.

21 "Comfort Mission Shows Renewed MHS Humanitarian Focus," Department of Defense, Force Health Protection & Readiness, accessed June 1, 2010, at http://intlhealth.fhpr.osd.mil/newsID112.mil.aspx.

22 Peter Hilsenrath, "Health Policy as Counter-Terrorism: Health Services and the Palestinians," *Defense and Peace Economics* 16, no. 5 (2005): 365–74, accessed June 2, 2010, at www.econpapers.repec.org/article/tafdefpea/v_3a16_3ay_3a2005_3ai_3a5_3ap_3a365-374.htm, doi: 10.1080/10242690500210831.

23 Harley Felbaum, *US Global Health and National Security Policy* (Washington, DC: CSIS, 2009).

Chapter 5. The Fox and the Hydra

1 Reuben Kessel, "Price Discrimination in Medicine," *Journal of Law and Economics* 1 (October 1958): 20–53.

2 Andrew H. Beck, "Medical Education: The Flexner Report and the Standardization of American Medical Education," *Journal of the American Medical Association* 291, no. 17 (2004): 2139–40.

3 Mark Harrison, *The Economics of World War II: Six Great Powers in International Comparison* (Cambridge: Cambridge University Press, 1998).

4 Charles Shrader, *History of Operations Research in the United States Army, Vol. 1: 1942–1962* (Washington, DC: US Army Center of Military History, 2006).

5 "Scientific Manpower Studies," National Science Foundation, accessed October 1, 2009, www.nsf.gov/pubs/1953/annualreports/ar_1953_sec4.pdf.

6 Ok Pannenborg, former Lead Health Advisory, World Bank, personal communication, October 21, 2010.

7 F. Mullan et al., "Results of the Sub-Saharan Medical School Study," *Lancet* 377 (November 20, 2010): 1113–21.

8 *Financing the Response to AIDS in Low- and Middle-Income Countries: International Assistance from the G8, European Commission and Other Donor Governments in 2008* (New York: UNAIDS/The Henry J. Kaiser Foundation, July 2010).

9 UNAIDS, *Report on the Global AIDS Epidemic* (Geneva: UNAIDS, 2008).

10 "PEPFAR Funding: Investments That Save Lives and Promote Security," PEPFAR, accessed October 4, 2011, at www.pepfar.gov/press/80064.htm.

11 Josephine Katabaazi Nakyanzi, Freddy Eric Kitutu, Hussein Oria, and Pakoyo Fadhiru Kamba, "Expiry of Medicines in Supply Outlets in Uganda," *Bulletin of the World Health Organization* 88 (2010): 154–58.

12 "PEPFAR Funding: Investments That Save Lives and Promote Security," PEPFAR, accessed October 4, 2011, at www.pepfar.gov/press/80064.htm.

Chapter 6. Successful Efforts to Curb Insourcing

1 Suwit Wibulpolprasert, "International Trade and Migration of Health Workforce: Experience from Thailand," paper presented at the Joint WTO World Bank Symposium of the Movement of Persons under GATS, WTO, Geneva, April 11–12, 2002.

2 Ibid.

3 Suwit Wibulpolprasert and Paichit Pengpaibon, "Integrated Strategies to Tackle the Inequitable Distribution of Doctors in Thailand: Four Decades of Experience," *Human Resources for Health* 1, no. 12 (2003), www.human-resources-health.com/content/1/1/12, doi:10.1186/1478-4491-1-12.

4 Nigel Hawkes, "NHS Closes Its Doors to Foreign Doctors," *Sunday Times* (London), February 8, 2008, www.timesonline.co.uk/tol/news/politics/article3321919.ece.

5 M. R. Schwartz, "The Physician Pipeline to Rural and Underserved Areas in Pennsylvania," *Journal of Rural Health* 24, no. 4 (Fall 2008): 384–89.

6 T. J. Mathews and Marian MacDorman, "Infant Mortality Statistics from the 2005 Period: Linked Birth/Infant Death Data Set," *National Vital Statistics Reports* 57, no. 2 (July 30, 2008), www.cdc.gov/nchs/data/nvsr/nvsr57/nvsr57_02.pdf.

7 Michelle Chen, "Death by Birth: Race and Maternal Mortality,"

Colorlines, March 16, 2010, http://colorlines.com/archives/2010/03/death_by_birth_race_and_maternal_mortality.html.

8 "Enriching Medicine through Diversity," American Medical Student Association, accessed November 18, 2009, at www.amsa.org/AMSA/Homepage/About/Mission/StrategicPriorities/EnrichingMedicineThroughDiversity.aspx.

Chapter 7. The Way Forward

1 Julio Frenk et al., "Health Professionals for a New Century: Transforming Education to Strengthen Health Systems in an Interdependent World," *Lancet* 376, no. 9756 (December 4, 2010): 1923–58, doi:10.1016/S0140-6736(10)61854-5.

2 "Cost-Effectiveness of Nurse Practitioners," World of Nurse Practitioners, accessed November 10, 2009, at www.worldofnursepractitioners.com/nurse-practitioner-cost-effectiveness.html.

3 "The Key to Making Lasting Lifestyle and Behavioral Changes: Is It Will or Skill?," American Psychological Association, accessed October 10, 2009, at www.apa.org/helpcenter/lifestyle-behavior.aspx.

4 "Physician Health Workforce Report," Bureau of Health Professions Research, accessed November 29, 2009, at http://bhpr.hrsa.gov/healthworkforce/reports/physicianworkforce/minority.htm.

5 H. K. Rabinowitz, J. J. Diamond, M. Hojat, and C. E. Hazelwood, "Demographic, Educational and Economic Factors Related to Recruitment and Retention of Physicians in Rural Pennsylvania," *Journal of Rural Health* 15, no. 2 (Spring 1999): 212–18.

6 Pamela S. Whitten et al., "Systematic Review of Cost Effectiveness Studies of Telemedicine Interventions," *British Medical Journal* 324 (2002): 1434.

7 F. M. Trevino, "The Representation of Hispanics in the Health Professions," *Journal of Allied Health* (Spring 1994): 65–77; M. Komaromy et al., "The Role of Black and Hispanic Physicians in Providing Health Care for Underserved Populations," *New England Journal of Medicine* 334, no. 20 (1996): 1305–10.

8 *Changing Demographics: Implications for Physicians, Nurses, and Other Health Workers* (Washington, DC: Bureau of Health Professions Research, 2003).

9 "Six-Year Medical Students Learning in a Hurry to Heal," Associated Press, accessed November 12, 2009, at www.sptimes.com/2004/12/05/Worldandnation/Six_year_medical_stud.shtml.

10 Katherine Mangan, "New Medical School Programs Put Students on a Fast Track to the White Coat," *Chronicle of Higher Education*, February 2, 2009.

11 J. S. Felton, "Burnout as a Clinical Entity—Its Importance in Health Care Workers," *Occupational Medicine*, December 4, 1997, http://occmed.oxfordjournals.org/content/48/4/237.abstract.

12 Rob Elgie, "Politics, Economics, and Nursing Shortages: A Look at U.S. Policies: Alternatives," MedScape, accessed November 19, 2009, at www.medscape.com/viewarticle/565608_9.

13 "Ethical Nurse Recruitment Position Statement," ICN, accessed November 8, 2010, at www.icn.ch/psrecruit01.htm.

14 "Code of Conduct for the Recruitment of Foreign Educated Nurses," American Nurses Association, accessed November 24, 2009, at www.nursingworld.org/MainMenuCategories/ThePracticeofProfessionalNursing/workplace/ForeignNurses/CodeofConductforRecruitmentofForeignEducatedNurses.aspx.

Index

AAMC (Association of American Medical Colleges), 19, 21, 30–31, 59–60
abuse of foreign-trained healthcare workers, 72, 172–174
Academic Ranking of World Universities, 40
Academy Health, 85
accreditation, 103–104
Accreditation Council for Graduate Medical Education, 21–22
admissions system in medical schools, 59–61
advanced-practice nurses, xiv–xv, 61–63, 154–155, 157
Afghanistan, healthcare as security issue in, 114
African Americans, 4, 49–50, 108–112, 119, 146–148, 159
African Health Workforce Program (World Bank), xx–xxi
aging: of baby boomers, 5, 18–19, 23; of nurses, 22–24; of patients, 18–19; of pharmacists, 24–25; of physicians, 19–22; of public-health and safety workers, 25–27. *See also* healthcare workers, aging of
AHECs (Area Health Education Centers), 148
alignment of student recruitment and training with healthcare needs, 158–160
Allied Health Professional Personnel Act (PL-751, 1966), 122
AMA (American Medical Association), 30–31, 118, 120
ambulatory care sensitive conditions, 36
American Academy of Pediatrics, xvi
American Association of Colleges of Nursing, 54, 57
American Association of Colleges of Pharmacy, 25
American Association of International Healthcare Recruitment, 173
American Association of Physicians of Indian Origin, 98
American Medical Association (AMA), 30–31, 118, 120
AMN Healthcare, 80
anthrax letters, 25–26
Apollo Hospital Systems, 93
applicability of foreign-acquired medical knowledge, 97
Area Health Education Centers (AHECS), 148

Aspen Institute, 135
associate-degree nursing programs, 55–56
Association of American Medical Colleges (AAMC), 19, 21, 30–31, 59–60
Association of Pakistani Physicians of North America, 98
asthma, 36
audiologists, 54–55, 163
autism, 29
avian flu, 27, 112

baby boomers, 5, 18–19, 23
Bachelet, Michelle, 104
bachelor of science in nursing, 55–56
Baker, Tim, xiv
Barbados, HIV/AIDS in, xviii–xx
behavior-change professions, 156–158
Bernard Hodes Group, 23
Bill and Melinda Gates Foundation, 130, 135
biochemists, 25
biomedical industry, 162
Bologna Process on Higher Education (European Commission), 136
bonding, 167–168
Botswana, HIV/AIDS in, 127
breach of contract fees, 84
British Department for International Development (DFID), 135
Brown Report (Carnegie Foundation), 52
Buerhaus, Peter, 23
bureaucracy. *See* international healthcare labor market regulation; regulation of healthcare workers
Bureau of Health Professions, 171–172, 173–174
Bureau of Primary Health Care, 160
Burkina Faso, healthcare worker shortage in, 95
burnout, 170
Bush, George W., 3, 113, 128

Canada, healthcare in, 35–36
Caribbean, HIV/AIDS in, xviii–xx
Carnegie Foundation, 48–49, 52, 118
Carroll Hospital Center, xviii
Carter, Jimmy, 120
CDC Epidemic Intelligence Service, 26
Cedar Crest College, 148–149
Center for Strategic International Studies, 114
Centers for Medicare and Medicaid Services (CMS), 14, 61
central-planning boards, 122–123
CGFNS (Commission on Graduates of Foreign Nursing Schools), 2–3, 74
child and infant mortality, xv–xvi, 4, 8, 15, 95, 125, 140–141, 146
China, nursing schools in, 2–3
Chopra, Deepak, 93
circular migration, 96–97

Cleveland Clinic, 170
clinical associates, 149
clinical rotations, 145
CMS (Centers for Medicare and Medicaid Services), 14, 61
Commission on Graduates of Foreign Nursing Schools (CGFNS), 2–3, 74
Commonwealth Code of Practice for the International Recruitment of Health Workers, 133
communication: about fatal diagnoses, 16; between healthcare workers, 13; with patients, 16–18
competition: among healthcare training providers, 117; among recruiting companies, 76, 80; fear of, 124; for healthcare workers, 37–39; for medical school entrance, 69
contracts for foreign workers, 76–78, 83–84, 174
Cooper, Richard "Buz," 38
costs, healthcare related: of healthcare worker shortage, 37; of healthcare worker training, 44–48, 50–59, 61–65, 126–127, 148–149, 155–156, 161–167; of insourcing, 2–3; of remittances, 106–107; of research, 162
Council on Medical Education (AMA), 49
Council on Physician and Nurse Supply, 24
credential creep, 40, 54–59, 163
credentialing, 81
Cross Country Staffing, 80
cultural competence, 6, 15–18, 112
culture of leaving, 102
cycled migration, 177–178

DB Healthcare, 79
debt, educational, 5, 46, 48, 55, 57, 62, 109–110, 164
Delaware, healthcare worker training in, 145
dengue fever, 112
dental HPSAs, 20
Department of Health, Education, and Welfare, 120
Department of Health and Human Services (HHS), 20, 22, 42, 120, 160, 171–172
Department of State Office of Private Sector Exchange, 88
dependent visas, 88
DFID (British Department for International Development), 135
diabetes, 4, 11, 18, 30, 36–37, 111, 156–157
diarrhea, 99–100
diploma nursing programs, 55–56
direct model of nurse recruitment, 78–79
disciplinary actions, physician, 72–73
doctors. *See* physicians
Doctors of Osteopathy (DOs), 163
Dr. Charles Brimm Medical Arts High School, 147
dropouts, 169–170

early retirement, 169–170
Ebola virus, 112
ECFMG (U.S. Education Commission for Foreign Medical Graduates), 103–104
Educational Commission for Foreign Medical Graduates, 71–72
educational debt, 5, 46, 48, 55, 57, 62, 109–110, 164
educational visas, 88
effective demand, 127
Eisenhower, Dwight D., 120
El Salvador, emigration from, 108
emergency code, 14
emergency room care, 35–37
English competency, 16–18
environmental-health workers, 27
Epidemic Intelligence Service, CDC, 26
epidemiologists, 25, 27
errors, medical, 11–13, 15, 58, 63
ethical lapses, physician, 73
Ethiopia, healthcare worker shortage in, 7, 91–92
Ethiopian North American Health Professionals Association, 98
European Community licensing of healthcare workers, 136
evidence-based recruitment and admissions, 158–160
Exchange Visitor Program, 88

family-health workers, 142
fatal diagnoses, communication about, 16
federal bonding, 167–168
feminization of medical profession, 22
Findley, Kathy, 165
flexible scheduling, 170
Flexner, Abraham, 49, 119–120
Flexner Report (Carnegie Foundation), 48–49, 119–121
FMG America, 70–71
foreign-trained healthcare workers: abuse of, 72, 172–174; contract process for, 76–78, 83–84, 174; cultural competence of, 6, 15–18, 112; English competency of, 16–18; grievance process for, 174; qualification and orientation of, 4. *See also* international recruitment industry; visas
foundations, healthcare, 134–135
free-market approach to international healthcare regulation, 118–121, 123–127
funding of healthcare worker training, 9, 38–39, 45, 51, 134–135, 145–146, 154, 164–167, 178–179
funeral directors, 17–18

GATS (General Agreement on Trade in Services), 136–137
gauze ceiling, 110
Geller, Colonel Dr. Schuyler K., 115
General Agreement on Trade in Services (GATS), 136–137
German Organization for Technical Cooperation, 135

Ghana, healthcare worker shortage in, 92
GHWA (Global Health Workforce Alliance), 9, 130–132
Global Health Workforce Alliance (GHWA), 9, 130–132
globalization of healthcare labor markets, impact of, 91–115; on health-education institutions in home countries, 101–104; on health in home countries, 94–101; overview, 91–94; on society in home countries, 104–108; on U.S. minorities and communities, 108–112; on U.S. security, 112–115
Global Law Center, 79
Global Universities Rankings, 40
Gore, Al, 113
green cards, 83
grievance process, 174
Guevara, Che, 105
guild-led regulation, 120–121

H-1B visas, 87, 89
H-1C visas, 87
Habte, Demissie, xx
Haiti, U.S. military response to 2010 earthquake, 114
Hart-Celler Immigrant Act (1965), 87
"Health as a Bridge to Peace and Stability" symposium, 115
healthcare regulatory system, international. *See* international healthcare labor market regulation
healthcare-related costs. *See* costs, healthcare related
healthcare-specific visas, 1, 3, 5–6, 10, 67, 106
healthcare worker associations, 124
healthcare worker density, 95
healthcare worker education fund (proposed), 166
healthcare workers: communication between, 13; competition for, 37–39; job-growth rate of, 38; licensing of, 54–59, 136; minority under-representation of, 108–112; overregulation of, 124; part-time, 170–171; productivity of, 168–171; retraining of, 124–127; self-regulation of, 121; understaffing of, 4; unemployment of, 105; unionization of, 5. *See also* foreign-trained healthcare workers; regulation of healthcare workers
healthcare workers, aging of, 10–39; and aging patients, 18–19; and competition for workers, 37–39; and emergency room care, 35–37; and health insurance reform, 30–32; and medically underserved areas, 32–34; nurses, 22–24; overview, 5, 10–18; pharmacists, 24–25; physicians, 19–22; public health and safety workers, 25–27; and technological advances, 27–30

healthcare workers, self-sufficiency of, 150–179; by aligning student recruitment and training with healthcare needs, 158–160; by increasing healthcare worker productivity, 168–171; by opening up federal bonding, 167–168; by over-hauling funding for training, 164–167; overview, 150–151; by rationalizing healthcare labor market, 171–172; by reducing training costs, 161–163; by regulation of foreign health-care recruitment, 172–179; by training more behavior-change healthcare workers, 156–158; by training more healthcare workers, 151–153; by training more midlevel providers, 154–156; by training more primary-care workers, 153–154

healthcare worker shortage, origins of, 40–65; accreditation of medical schools, 61–63; admissions system in medical schools, 59–61; and credential creep, 40; funding of, foreign, 54–59; medical training, high cost of, 44–48; and nursing education, 51–59; overview, xxi–xxii, 40–41; public vs. private medical schools, 63–65; and regulation, 41–45; research, emphasis on, 48–51

healthcare worker training: costs of, 44–48, 50–59, 61–65, 126–127, 148–149, 155–156, 161–167; funding of, 9, 38–39, 45, 51, 134–135, 145–146, 154, 164–167, 178–179; funding of, foreign, 102, 125; impact of emigration on, 101–104; lack of access to, 6; nurses, 51–59; outsourcing of, 63–64; in Pennsylvania, 143–146; physicians, 44–51; public vs. private, 63–65; reducing insourcing by reducing training costs, 148–149; in research-oriented universities, 48–54; in rural areas, 143–146; for self-sufficiency, 151–163; short-term, 124–127; standards for, 137

health insurance: payment differentials, 154; and preventive care, 158; universal, 35–36

health insurance reform, 30–32

Health Professional Shortage Areas (HPSAs), 20

Health Profession Council of South Africa, 104

Health Resources and Services Administration (HRSA), 24, 171

HealthSouth, 29

Health Status and Health Care Access of Farm and Rural Populations (USDA), 33

Health Workforce Unit (WHO), 129–131

heath insurance reform, 30–34

Helping Babies Breathe, xvi

HHS. *See* Department of Health and Human Services (HHS)
Hispanic-Serving Institutions (HSIs), 148
Historically Black Colleges and Universities, 148
HIV/AIDS, xviii–xx, 112–113, 127–133
homosexuality, 15–16
Hope Street Group, xxi–xxii
Howard University, 148
HPSAs (Health Professional Shortage Areas), 20
HRSA (Health Resources and Services Administration), 24, 171
HSIs (Hispanic-Serving Institutions), 148

IMG Digest, 72
immigration-law firms, 79
India, healthcare worker shortage in, 93–94
India, HIV/AIDS in, 127
infant mortality, xv–xvi, 4, 8, 15, 95, 125, 140–141, 146
infectious-disease specialists, 26
insourcing, defined, 1
insourcing, successful efforts to curb, 138–149; in minority communities, 146–148; overview, 138–140; Philippines, 140–141; by reducing training costs, 148–149; Sri Lanka, 141–142; United Kingdom, 142–143; United States, 143–146
insurance. *See* health insurance
international accreditation, 103–104
International Council of Nurses, 82, 172
international healthcare labor market regulation, 116–137; efforts to correct, 132–137; free-market, post–World War II, 123–127; free-market, pre–World War II, 118–121; by international and bilateral organizations, 127–132; manpower planning during World War II, 121–123; organizations capable of addressing, 134–135; overview, 116–118
International Labor Organization, 134
International Medical Graduates Advisors Network, 72
international nurse-recruitment industry, 73–80
International Organization for Migration, 134
international physician-recruitment industry, 68–73
international recruitment industry, 66–90; nurse recruitment, 73–76; nurse recruitment as big business, 76–80; overview, 66–68; physician recruitment, 68–73; recruitment-agency services, 80–82; selling visas instead of training workers, 86–90; staffing agencies,

84–86; unethical recruiting practices, 70–71, 82–84
IntraHealth International, 135
IT (information technology) recruiting companies, 79–80

J-1 Visitor Exchange Program (J-1 visas), 88–89
JAMA (*Journal of the American Medical Association*), 12, 50
Jamaica: healthcare as security issue in, 114; nurse-vacancy rate in, 7
Japanese International Cooperation Agency (JICA), 135
JCAHO (Joint Commission on Accreditation of Healthcare Organizations), 12
Jefferson Medical College, Thomas Jefferson University, 144
JICA (Japanese International Cooperation Agency), 135
John D. and Catherine T. MacArthur Foundation, 135
Johns Hopkins University School of Medicine, 50–51, 152
Johns Hopkins University School of Nursing, 152
Joint Commission of Accreditation of Healthcare Organizations (JCAHO), 12, 173
Journal of the American Medical Association (*JAMA*), 12, 50

Kaiser Family Foundation, 25
Kemp, Stephen, 17–18
Kenya, healthcare worker shortage in, 107
know/do gap, 125

labor-market dropouts, 169–170
lab technicians, xiv, 27, 110
language barriers, 16–18
Latino access to healthcare and healthcare training, 108–112, 146–148, 159–160
Latino immigrants, 107–108
LCME (Liaison Committee on Medical Education), 42, 61–63, 103
legal liability, 85
Lesotho, healthcare worker shortage in, 100–101
Liaison Committee on Medical Education (LCME), 42, 61–63, 103
licensed practical nurses, 74, 81, 84, 169
license revocations, physician, 72–73
licensing of healthcare workers, 54–59, 136
long-term nursing homes, 14

malaria, 112
Malawi: healthcare educator shortage in, 101; healthcare worker shortage in, 92–93, 107
Mali, healthcare worker shortage in, 94
malpractice insurance, 171
manpower planning, 121–123
manpower studies, 121

Marburg virus, 112–113
Mary's Center for Maternal and Child Health, xvii
Massachusetts health insurance reform, 31–32
maternal mortality, 91, 95, 141, 146
MCAT (Medical College Admission Test), 59–60
Medicaid, 45, 61, 85
Medical College Admission Test (MCAT), 59–60
medical education. *See* healthcare worker training
Medical Education in the United States and Canada. See Flexner Report (Carnegie Foundation)
medical errors, 11–13, 15, 58, 63
medically complex children, 29
medically underserved areas, 32–34, 89–90
medical schools: accreditation of, 61–63; impact of Flexner Report on, 48–51, 120
Medicare, 33, 45, 61, 85, 122, 173
mental-health HSPAs, 20
Merlin, 135
Merritt Hawkins & Associates, 19, 34
micro-preemies, 29
midcareer healthcare students, 165
midlevel healthcare providers, 154–156
midwives, 99, 154–156
Military Accessions Vital to National Interest, 86–87
minorities in U.S.: impact of Flexner Report on, 119; impact of healthcare worker insourcing on, 108–112; in medically underserved areas, 32–34, 89–90; successful efforts to curb insourcing, 146–148
molecular biologists, 25–26
monitoring and evaluation (M&E) experts, xx
Morrow, Richard, xiv

National Council Licensure Examination (NCLEX), 74–75, 81
National Council of State Nursing Boards, 172
National Health Service (U.K.), 103–104, 142–143
National Health Service Corps, 167–168
National Health Workforce Commission, 172
National Hospital Association, 172
National Resident Matching Program, 68–70
Native American access to healthcare and healthcare training, 146, 148, 159–160
NCLEX (National Council Licensure Examination), 74–75, 81
negligence, 14
New England Journal of Medicine, 13
NGOs focusing on healthcare, 135

"no beds available," 33–34
Norwegian Agency for Development Cooperation, 135
nurse educators, 53–54, 148–149, 152
nurse practitioners, xiv, 57, 122, 154–156, 163
nurses: advanced-practice, xiv–xv; aging of, 22–24; and breach of contract fees, 84; education of, 51–59; international recruitment of, 67, 73–80; licensed practical, 74, 81, 84, 169; nurse's aides, 169; recruitment-agency services for, 80–82; staffing ratios, 15; striking of, 15; substandard wages for, 83; turnover rate, 13; understaffing of, 14–15; unethical recruiting practices, 82–84
nurse's aides, 169
nurse-to-patient ratios, Medicare and Medicaid, 85
"Nursing for the Future" (Carnegie Foundation), 52
nursing homes, long-term, 14
Nursing Relief for Disadvantaged Areas Act (1999), 87

Obama, Barack, 2, 113–114
obesity, 30, 111
occupational therapists, 24, 55, 121
Office of Private Sector Exchange, Department of State, 88
older healthcare students, 165
orientation for foreign workers, 175
osteopathic medicine, 162–163
outsourcing of healthcare worker training, 63–64
overregulation, 124
overspecialization, 46

Palestinian territories, healthcare as security issue in, 114
parent shifts, 170
part-time healthcare workers, 170–171
Patient Protection and Affordable Care Act, 30–31
patients, aging of, 18–19
pediatrics, 29, 33, 35, 68, 154–155, 166, 170, 175
Pennsylvania, healthcare worker training in, 143–146
pent-up unmet medical needs, 31–32
PEPFAR (President's Emergency Plan for AIDS Relief), 113, 128, 133
Perry, Rick, 161
Peters, David, 131
pharmacists, 24–25, 133
Philippines, successful efforts to curb insourcing in, 140–141
phlebotomists, xiv, 110
Phoya, Ann, 74
physical therapists, 55, 88, 163
physician assistants, xiv, 122, 154–156
physicians: aging of, 19–22; average workweek for, 21–22;

disciplinary actions on, 72–73; Doctors of Osteopathy, 163; education of, 44–51; ethical lapses by, 73; impact of Flexner Report on, 120; international recruitment of, 67–73; license revocations of, 72–73; as most educated citizens, 104–105; pediatrics, 29, 33, 35, 68, 154–155, 166, 170, 175; physician-to-population ratio, 19–20; primary-care, 21, 28, 31–33, 35–37, 46, 62, 120; resident, 21–22, 39, 68–70; women, 22
Physicians for Human Rights, 130
Physician Shortage Area Program (PSAP), 144–145
placement fees, 81
placement model of nurse recruitment, 76–77
Pleasant Care Corporation, 14
Preker, Alex, 102
premature babies, 29
President's Emergency Plan for AIDS Relief (PEPFAR), 113–114, 128, 133
preventive care, 156–158
primary-care physicians, 21, 28, 31–33, 35–37, 46, 62, 120
primary-care workers, 4, 12, 20–21, 46, 57, 153–154
private vs. public healthcare education, 63–65, 122, 141
productivity of healthcare workers, 168–171
professional elitism, 50
PSAP (Physician Shortage Area Program), 144–145
public-health communication experts, 26
public-health workers, 25–27
public-safety workers, 25–27
public vs. private healthcare education, 63–65, 122, 141

quarantine officers, 27

radiation-health experts, 26
rationalization of healthcare labor market, 171–172
rationing of healthcare, 34
ratios: nurse-to-patient, Medicare and Medicaid, 85; physician-to-population, 19–20; primary-care physicians to specialists, 21; staffing, 15
recommendations for healthcare worker self-sufficiency. *See* healthcare workers, self-sufficiency of recruitment-agency services, 80–82
registered nurses. *See* nurses
regulation of healthcare workers, 21–22, 41–45, 62–63, 116, 120–121, 163, 172–179. *See also* international healthcare labor market regulation
remittances, 106–108
research: as driver of healthcare training costs, 162; and medical education, 48–51; and nursing education, 51–54

resident physicians, 21–22, 39, 68–70
retraining of healthcare workers, 124–127
return service, 167
Rockefeller Foundation, 135
Rosenthal, Eric, 165–166
Rotary Foundation, 135
rural areas, access to healthcare, 32–34, 44, 89–90, 143–146, 159–160
Rural Medicine program, 148

salmonella, 26
SARS, 27, 112
Save the Children, 135
Schedule A shortage occupations, 88–89
schedule flexibility, 170
schistosomiasis, 98
security impact of global healthcare. *See* globalization of healthcare labor markets, impact of SEIU (Service Employees International Union), 172
self-regulation, 121
self-sufficiency of healthcare workers. *See* healthcare workers, self-sufficiency of
seniors: communication with foreign healthcare workers, 17; healthcare needs of, 18–19; hospitalization rates of, 19; and language barriers, 17; and technological advances, 28–29
Sentosa Recruitment Agency, 84
Service Employees International Union (SEIU), 172
sexual history, patient's, 16
short-term training of healthcare workers, 124–127
Singh, Manmohan, 93
Siskind Susser, 79
social impact of healthcare worker emigration, 104–108
social sensitivity. *See* cultural competence
South Africa, healthcare worker shortage in, 103–104
Spelman College, 148
Sri Lanka, successful efforts to curb insourcing in, 141–142
staffing agencies, 84–86
staffing model of nurse recruitment, 77–78
staffing ratios, 15
standardization of medical education, 48–49, 137
Stevens, Barbara, 165–166
stress-reduction programs, 170
strikes, nursing, 15
swine flu, 27

technological advances, 27–30
telemedicine, 160
Tennessee Institutes for Pre-Professionals (TIP), 147
terrorism, 12, 113–114
Test of English as a Foreign Language (TOEFL), 16–17
Thailand, healthcare workers in, 138–140
Thomas Jefferson University, 144